Hope in the Hard Places:

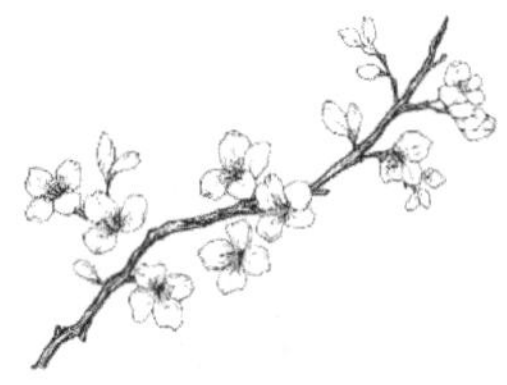

My Journey through the Devastation of Lyme Disease

By Erika Goering

ISBN: 9798884535763

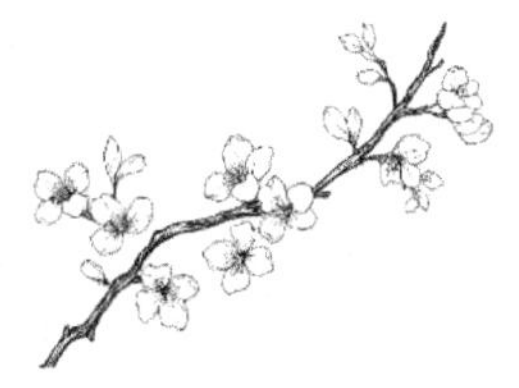

YOU NEVER KNOW HOW STRONG YOU ARE
UNTIL BEING STRONG IS THE ONLY CHOICE
YOU HAVE.

-BOB MARLEY-

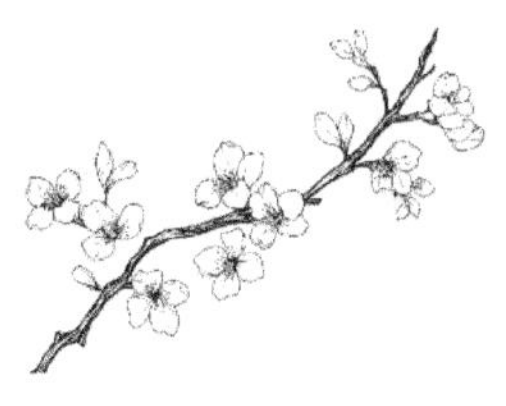

CONTENTS

ACKNOWLEDGMENTS — i

DEDICATION — iii

INTRODUCTION — 1

CHAPTER 1 — 11

CHAPTER 2 — 26

CHAPTER 3 — 36

CHAPTER 4 — 41

CHAPTER 5 — 48

CHAPTER 6 — 56

CHAPTER 7 — 64

CHAPTER 8 — 76

CHAPTER 9 — 85

ABOUT THE AUTHOR — 100

RESOURCES — 102

   GENERAL PRODUCTS — 102

   YOUNG LIVING PRODUCTS — 103

   PROVIDERS — 105

   LYME ARTICLES — 105

   CONNECT WITH ME — 106

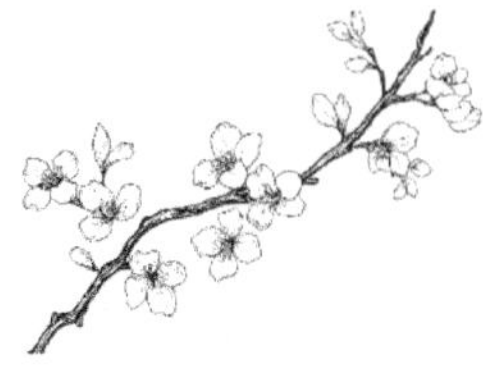

ACKNOWLEDGMENTS

There would not be a book if it weren't for my children. I will never forget the drive home from swim team when you spoke life into me. You were watching and learning from all that I went through, and you were the ones who cast my vision for this book. You never allowed me to quit when the writing became overwhelming. You cheered for me from the first evening until the moment this book was complete.

Thank you to Wendy Speake for listening to my visions of a book draft and knowing where to point me. Watching you share your stories and then placing them in book form inspired me that I could do it too. You were the one to point me to the editor. Your ability to listen and speak truth into a soul was the wind beneath my wings at the right moment.

Thank you to Bethany for reading my first version of the book and ever so graciously helping with the editing. Your gentle guidance and commitment to crafting a book that would reach the right audience came into my life at the perfect time.

Liz, you came along to take me to the finish line. I don't take it for granted that you have an appreciation and understanding of the natural world of health and wellness. Thank you for the numerous phone calls, texts for encouragement, and multiple emails making sure that I finished the adventure of writing my first book.

Lisa, I'm forever grateful to you for the time you and our family have spent in your office. Thank you for the very first phone call while I was in Japan. You heard the desperation in my voice. You felt the pain and agony that I had been through and understood my feelings of hopelessness. I knew I was in good hands when our first meeting began with a long embrace. Thank you for not just helping me with my health, but for caring even more for my spirit. Your shared tears let me know that your care went far beyond just the health advice and help you gave me. You are a huge part of my story and without you in it, this story could have ended a whole lot differently.

Michele, you are a true gem of a friend. It takes a certain kind of friend to patiently introduce me to a whole new way of living. You were ever so gracious as you opened my eyes to the world of coffee enemas, cooked veggie recipes, hair analysis, and supplements to support my journey. I'm forever grateful that God brought you back to Japan for such a time as this. I needed the information that you had. Thank you!

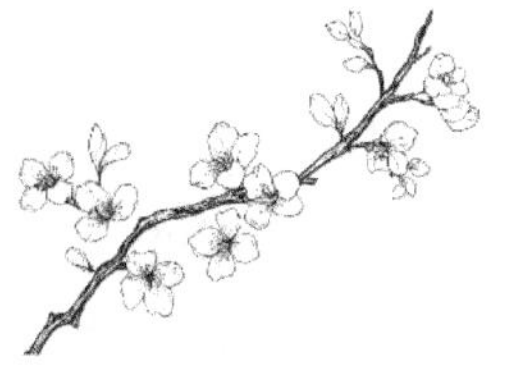

DEDICATION

I would like to acknowledge that without the support of numerous friends and family, our journey would have looked much different. Without the meals, car rides, deliveries, cleaners, parties, and so much more, the three years of what seemed like darkness would have been much darker. You were the lights in our dark season. You were the perfect phone call at just the right moment. You were the ones who answered endless texts asking for prayers, support, urgent needs, and more. You heard my fears and listened while I cried. You pointed my thoughts back to the One who created me. You challenged me to think bigger and to never give up. From birthday cakes to laying your hands on me and praying, you were the hands and feet of our Father, and we are forever grateful.

My four children saw it all. I do not doubt that they are left with scars that only our Father can heal. You, dear ones, were the reason I fought so hard. I knew you deserved my best because in this season of sickness, each one of our hearts was challenged and bruised. Each of us was longing for something better. But for so many reasons, and for many we will never understand, our God allowed this season to occur. Every single day, my biggest prayer was for my healing. I knew that you needed me. I could apologize for all of it, but I know that my sickness wasn't my fault, nor was it yours. If I could go back and erase these years of illness, I would do so in a heartbeat. There were days when you were home alone wondering if your mom was going to live. There were nights when you had to put yourselves to sleep. There were games, birthdays, and school days that you went through without me cheering you on and celebrating you. I am sorry. I have to trust that this didn't just happen to me, but to all of us, and that there was a purpose in all of it for each of us. May your characters be stronger. May your faith be deeper. May your knowledge of your body and its ability to heal itself be richer. May your dependence on our Savior be what shines through your story. This is part of your story too, and I write this so that you too will remember the journey and how and WHO carried you through. I am better because of you. Each of you watched as I became healthier. You were the ones who cheered me on even in the darkest of days. I love you!

From the first night of my shaking hands, Brian was the one by my side. You, Babe, were the one who called the doctors. You fought for me when no one listened. You made endless phone calls when we couldn't get answers. You believed in me, and you never once doubted me. You heard my cries of fear and pain in the darkest of nights. You drove me to the appointments and advocated for me when I had nothing left to give. When the pain was too great, you prayed, covered me in oils, and massaged my back until I could relax enough to find rest. You had endless nights of no sleep, and yet you still got up and went to work. You were the one who carried me back and forth to the bathroom. You have humbled me by how graciously you cared for not only our children, but also by how you compassionately bathed me, dressed me, and so much more. You knew my fear of staying in a foreign hospital, so you never left my side. I not only fought for health because of the kids, but also because of you. I knew that you also deserved to live a healthy life with your spouse. We have far too many more adventures to live and pursue together. Thank you for believing in me when I decided to travel back to Japan and begin my healing journey. Thank you for tucking me back into bed and telling me that I would soon be better when I had not an ounce of faith left. Thank you for believing in and respecting my choice to pursue healing via the natural homeopathic way. Thank you for trusting me and my own judgement to seek the avenues that I felt led to pursue. I write this book so that we will never ever forget what God took us through. This chapter of our lives was a deep valley, but I am honored that we came out the other side stronger, more knowledgeable, and most of all, together. May we never ever forget where we have come from. I love you!

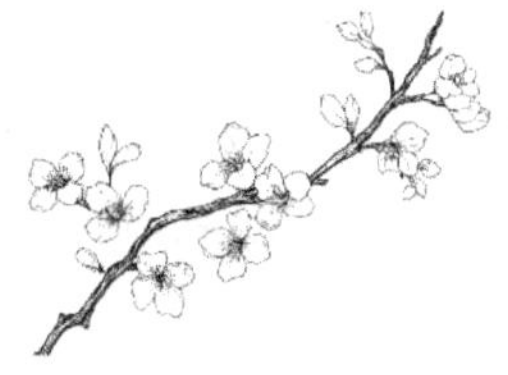

INTRODUCTION

Let's Get Acquainted

Hey there! Cozy up with your favorite beverage of choice, and let's chat. I wish with all my heart that I could sit next to you on your living room couch and hear every single detail of your story. Your story matters, and if you are reading this book, I'm gonna guess that your story ain't been easy. Mine wasn't an easy one either, but I fought Lyme disease, and now that I am on the other side, I want to share with you my journey in hopes that you find encouragement. If you were here with me, I would pull out the tissues, turn on the diffuser, share a beverage or snack with essential oils added, give you lots of hugs, and just listen.

First, let me introduce myself and tell you my hopes for you as you read this book. I am a California girl by birth, but I spent most of my childhood growing up in the Midwestern wheat fields. At the age of seven, I gave my first-grade teacher some serious concerns. She believed that I needed to repeat the first grade due to my lack of ability to meet her academic standards. My parents fought to move me forward, and I believe that experience was a defining moment in my life. My parents' tenacity taught me that I did have what it takes to journey forward; it just might take me a little longer, and I might have to work just a little harder. I also learned that I could do anything when others believed in me, but most of all, I had to believe in myself. Little did I know how much learning these lessons would teach me about fighting for health in my life. I'm a woman of serious grit and a whole lot of grace. Well . . . I'll admit that sometimes I might need a little more grace and a lot less grit.

I met my man at the ripe age of five years old, but it took him about twenty years to realize that I was his gift from the Lord. He then grabbed his guitar, sang me a song, broke the guitar strings, and pulled out a ring. At the young age of twenty-four, we tied the knot and headed south to Texas. Our Texas roots grew deep in the eight short years that we lived there, and we met friends that forever changed our hearts and lives.

During our time in Texas, the Lord grew us in ways that we never could have anticipated. We have seven kids total, four of them here in our home. Yes, we have experienced the loss of three children. Miscarriages and ectopic pregnancies are heartbreaking. We've been there, and we know the pain. We are now a family of six. We like to refer to ourselves as the 6G Network, 'cuz this mama thinks that sounds cool, but you should see the eye rolls from our teens.

INTRODUCTION

Nearly ten years ago, the Lord moved our family over the Pacific Ocean to Japan. Never did we have Japan on our list of places that we would dream of raising our kids, but the Lord always knows best. We took the leap of faith and threw caution to the wind because we wanted to show the kids a worldview that was larger than the state of Texas. Living on one fixed income as a teacher proved to be more than stressful. Sure, there are seriously challenging moments in raising kids overseas, but aren't there challenging moments raising kids anywhere? We could barely pay the bills, let alone take a vacation to the next county over. But, we knew that by living overseas there would be doors opened that we just could not provide if we stayed in America.

I will never forget the anxiety we felt as we said our farewells to our family and friends, but we also both had such peace, a peace that comes from knowing that you are walking in your purpose. Walking in what you are called to do can make others' heads spin, but we chose to walk in confidence as we embraced our family and friends and said goodbye. We had no idea what was ahead, but we knew that it had to be better than what we were leaving behind.

No one can prepare you for culture shock. You can study. You can do your best to learn the language and the culture, but it can't compare with actually being there. Besides, we only had a two-month warning to pack up and head out. Learning the culture wasn't as high on the list as spending as much time with the grandparents as possible, selling our belongings, scheduling packers, or learning a new job. Not only were we surrounded by the complexity of living in a new country, but we were also learning to embrace a differing sub-culture in our interactions with the military folks. It was a rough transition. I can pretty much sum it up with this: it was not pretty. There were high moments that took your breath away, but then there would be a low moment where you found yourself on the floor crying, wondering if you had just made the biggest mistake of your life. There were days when I did not speak English to anyone but our children. I longed for friends. I longed for one simple thing to prove itself easy. Everything took longer than expected, from going to the local grocery store and not knowing if you were buying the right diapers for your baby to realizing that the entire neighborhood now knows that you cannot separate trash according to their system because yours is the only one left sitting in the blazing sun after the trash man had already visited the neighborhood.

Assimilating into a foreign country and two different sub-cultures (the military and the Department of Defense) all at once proved to be completely exhilarating and yet absolutely exhausting. The theme song from the old TV show *Cheers* kept repeating over and over in my head: "Sometimes you wanna go where everybody knows your name." I longed for one familiar face who knew me well enough that even on my worst of days that friend would know, "Oh, she will be okay." Instead, I felt like my moments of meltdown proved me to be a crazy woman to the onlooking locals. New friendships do not happen overnight. Building friendships with others who don't speak the same language takes even longer. Time is what we needed. Acclimating to so many new cultures meant lots of transition. Time has proved to be a healing balm to huge moments of transition in my life, and time was what we all needed.

Apparently, extra time was something my husband and I had on our hands. I have type O-blood. Despite being cautioned not to conceive any more children while stationed in Japan because the Japanese don't stock a reliable surplus of my particular blood type, after a few short months in the country we found out that we were expecting our fourth child. God has a way of keeping us humble. I had made my own deal with God back when I had decided that thirty-five was a ripe old age to close up the womb and declare our family complete. Now God, on the other hand, knew better than I, and during the same week as I rang in my thirty-fifth birthday, He let us know that our family would be expanding.

What I have learned from numerous moves in twenty-one years of marriage is that a sense of normalcy in our new locations usually doesn't happen until experiencing an entire calendar year of holidays and seasons. During that year one, you adjust to new festivals, new places to shop for simple things like groceries, and new ways of celebrating holidays. After a year, we knew more of what to expect, how to embrace the culture, and how to navigate the little daily adventures of living in a foreign country.

Within a matter of about fourteen months our family experienced an overseas move, three different cultures, a literal tsunami, a hospitalization from strep, three cases of chicken pox, a new baby, giving birth far from home. It tested our family's faith in God, tenacity of spirit, grit for doing the hard, and flexibility of character. During this time, we also realized that our 900-square-foot house was not the most suitable location for a family of six, so we threw in a little more character testing and decided to move from the local town to the American-owned military base.

While laying our newborn baby down for a nap one afternoon, I was struck with the overwhelming realization that if our family hadn't already gone through such testing and refinement of our faith during our earlier years of marriage, I'm not sure that we would have been up for the challenges those fourteen months brought. Throughout these months there was so much undoing of our own expectations, stretching of beliefs, and opening of our eyes to a world bigger than ourselves. Numerous moments forced us to begin building a family that was strong enough to endure and even thrive, despite all of what others might have seen as chaos. Though this season of having four kids under the age of eight and showing them a whole new way of life proved to be more than we could handle on our own, the beautiful thing was that God brought us through it together as a couple and as a family.

I have been told a time or two that I am "bossy." I just like to think that I know what I want and how to get there. I am married to a man that knows what he wants, but he wants to make sure everyone is happy and peaceful in his pursuit of achieving his ways of getting there. He will also poll everyone's thoughts and do a ton of research before making a decision. I tend to jump from the plane, pray to God the parachute works, and maybe try to figure it out as I plummet to the ground. By God's grace we have enjoyed being married for almost twenty-three glorious years.

Never say never in life, because what I have found is those "never" statements usually turn into moments where I have to eat my words. Marrying the sexiest man from my hometown was one of those kinda moments. I never imagined marrying someone that I had grown up with, but somehow everyone else around us saw it coming. There are so many things that I appreciate about my man, but one thing that stands out to me is his willingness to learn, to stretch and be stretched in his mindset. Neither of us ever expected to be homeschooling our four kiddos, let alone be doing it in a foreign country. Neither of us had a clue about the more natural way of living and supporting our bodies until we nearly lost our three-year-old son to salmonella poisoning. But I didn't have to do it alone. Brian never let me stand alone in my pursuit of homeschooling or in my embracing the world of natural health.

Parenting and running our home have always been something that we have learned about and grown in together. So when I stood before him and declared that I thought that we were called to homeschool, and then later when I declared that I was ready to run my oils business, I knew that I would have 100% of his support, whether he knew all of the details or not. Marriage is oftentimes a balancing act, and ours certainly has been given my tendency to jump into something without knowing all of the details and his tendency to sit in front of the computer seeking out all of the current research first.

I always knew I would have a large family even from an early age. I also always cared about helping others learn; I am a teacher by trade who eventually went rogue and decided to homeschool. But natural health and essential oils becoming my jam came later in my life. Oils have completely changed the way that we run our home and our health, and sharing with my friends that they too can make these changes fills my cup to overflowing. Now, I not only find myself educating our children, but also teaching my friends, which keeps me doing what I am passionate about and at home with the kids. I believe that I am living the best of both worlds through adding to our family income and adding to the value of our children's education.

Health and wellness are my passion because they weave together mind, body, and spirit. Over and over in our lives, we have been challenged to seek research and grow our minds in the aspects of wellness. Our hearts have been shattered by a family suicide. Our bodies have been wrecked through the damaging effects of salmonella poisoning, Lyme disease, and depression. Our spirits have been broken down in moments of utter despair. However, we have also learned that there are numerous avenues to pursue when it comes to health and wellness. We have been forced to keep an open mind. We have learned the benefits of a really sound counselor, and we have also come to understand that our bodies were created to heal themselves. I have seen the beauty that comes from fighting for something truly worthwhile and the healing and restoration that can come after a long struggle.

I write this book to encourage you on so many fronts. You are not alone! All of the physical pains that you are feeling are real. The emotional effects of sickness can leave lasting wounds. But I have great news—we serve a God who desires to show you the road to wellness. Your journey will look different than mine, but I hope there are pieces of my story that you needed to hear, pieces that encourage you and some that you can identify with. Your journey is your own, but you are not alone. May the reading of this book deliver hope and inspire you to pursue wellness, because you are worth fighting for.

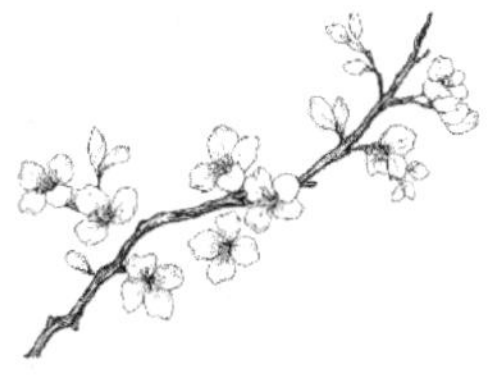

CHAPTER 1

Sickness

When I was young, forty years old seemed like it was lightyears away. Before I knew it though, life snuck up on me, and I found myself ringing in the beginning of the year by turning forty years old. Little did I know that this would be the year that would test just how much grit I truly had in me. Right around the time that I was celebrating forty years, I remember stepping out of the shower and noticing something that looked like a pimple on the side of my right rib cage. Thinking it was a weird place to have puss, I quickly released it, put my oils on, and then moved on. I did have a rash of redness around the area (not a bull's eye rash though), but it never looked like something to be too concerned about. No infection grew, but the wound was deep, and it left a scar.

Less than thirty days after the appearance of that strange pimple, I began to have uncontrollable shaking on my right side that started in my arm. Of course, the shaking scared me to death. I made my husband watch exactly what was going on, but we both had no idea what to think. He told me that maybe I was getting sick and that I should go to bed. I remember feeling exhausted, so I took his advice and went to bed and prayed to God for the shaking to stop.

The shaking went away for a few days, but when it came back, it was now uncontrollable on both sides of my body. As soon as I told my husband that I couldn't feel one side of my face, he got on the phone and called the emergency room. Living overseas presents a myriad of hurdles when it comes to doctors or emergency care. As Department of Defense workers, we had access to the on-base medical facilities with military medicine. In addition, we were allowed to seek care at the local hospitals and clinics. The choice is always up to us, but at this stage in our journey, we wanted to be able to communicate with our healthcare providers, so we chose to pursue providers who spoke our first language. The local on-base doctors recommended that I be seen, but they did confess that they didn't have any idea what was wrong with me. Since they had no idea what could be causing me to shake, we chose to not seek medical care and instead chose to pray, and of course, oil up. After that, I decided to go to bed and pray that the shaking would stop. When my body calmed, the shaking seemed to calm, but not for long.

In the middle of the night, I woke up because I could not catch my breath. I will never forget sitting straight up in bed and grasping my chest. I had been so thankful for the shaking to stop and even more thankful that I had able to go to sleep, but now my heart was pounding like I had just run a race. Forget the fact that I still couldn't feel the left side of my face because it had gone completely numb. I decided that maybe I was having a heart attack. Some people would want to say that it was anxiety, but the anxiety would come later.

It was the middle of the night, and we had four sleeping children and no one to just run over and watch them while we went to the doctor, so we did the only things we knew to do. We prayed like never before and used our toolbox of oils. As I lay there asking God to slow my breath and bring my racing heart back to a steady beat, I wondered if life as we once knew it was gone. What was happening to me? I was scared. I felt so alone. I wondered if my life was over. What brought me down to a calm that delivered sleep was my husband massaging my spine with oils and prayer. I had recently learned how powerful the oils that come from trees are, and I found that they quickly helped soothe my mind. Soon my breath returned, my heart found its rhythm, and I found the most important healing remedy: sleep.

Within the next few days, the severe abdominal pain began, and that is when I began to panic. My body seemed to be completely falling apart. Eating became very difficult, and my physical strength was waning. We did not want to ignore potential appendicitis, so my husband drove me to the emergency room. After hours and hours of waiting and testing, we were sent home with no answers. The MRI showed nothing in my body that would tell them why I was randomly shaking, having a racing heart, and now experiencing severe abdominal pain. How could someone be experiencing such random, seemingly-important symptoms, and yet no one could pinpoint the cause? I'm not sure that I have ever felt more alone in my life. It's a strange place to be when you are the only one who can feel the racing heart, the stabbing pain in the stomach, the gasping for air, the face that has no feeling, and all you see are eyes staring back at you with not one single real answer. We went home feeling completely hopeless, with anxious spirits and a new bag of stronger painkillers.

Taking that much medication did not solve any problems. It seemed to just add more. Each night, we prayed to God that our sleep would not be interrupted by the now nightly occurrence of my heart racing. But on one particular night, before my heart could awaken me, my insides woke me up with a bang. A bang! It wasn't a little pain. I truly felt an explosion inside of my body under my right rib cage. The explosion awakened me, and I bolted upright, screaming. I could feel it sending shrapnel all over my insides. The shaking began again, and the heart racing returned. One side of my brain began to tingle. We had no recourse, since the doctors had just told us that they could find nothing wrong with my body. So, we did what I'd done so many times: I rubbed oils and prayed until I could sleep.

The next day, I began to have extreme leg pain that started at my knees. Within days, the pain ran down to my feet, and it did not go away. On the days that my husband was at home, he would come and carry me from the bed to the tub so that I could bathe in essential oils to help remove the pain. On the days when it was just me and the kids, I spent most of the day in bed, and when I needed to move, crawling was the only way to get around. The oils that seemed to help the most in the bath were peppermint and wintergreen. I bathed numerous times a day, adding Epsom salt and essential oils to each bath. It was extremely humbling to need to be carried to the toilet and the tub! There were times when my left arm was completely numb, so my husband would have to help me pull up my pants when I got dressed. I would cry as I was carried. I was losing all sense of my independence. This was happening so quickly and without any answers. During these weeks, I learned that every time I ate, my stomach pains would worsen. Soon, I gave up on eating. I went days without eating much at all because it made the pain too unbearable.

My body was shutting down quite literally, but my spirit was also shutting down to the world. Friends would call or text to check in and see how they could pray or tangibly help. At times I avoided answering because I felt like silence was better than sharing the negative thoughts swirling in my head. In order for my mind and heart to cope, I withdrew from life and went inside of myself. The smile was gone from my face, and I became increasingly silent. The days began to run one into the other, and my soul began to feel hopeless.

At this point, my husband thought he was losing his wife, and to some degree he was. I could no longer take care of myself, and I still had four little ones who needed me. Our children were going through their own trauma of worrying about their mom, and yet none of us knew what to do or where to turn. My husband took so many days off work in order to care for me and our children. Eventually, he ran out of paid leave and had to return to work, so the kids and I found ourselves alone at home. I was the parent, and yet I found myself needing a parent of my own to help care for us. Our children had to rise to the challenge and run the home, and I knew they were hurting. They would come to my bedside with pictures that they had colored and cards of encouragement that they had written. They would prepare food for me and insist that I must eat it. Their schooling was suffering, and there was little I could do. We filled a basket of their books that made its home next to my bed. Each child would have their time next to me in the bed, and we would read and navigate any unfinished work together. There were numerous times that they would be reading to me and I would fall asleep. I had never been so tired in all of my life. I felt like a failure as a parent knowing that our children deserved better. They deserved a healthy mom. How was I going to get back my health? The testing of our character was being hit from all sides, and we were deep in the fight for the wellbeing of our family.

A loved one can only watch their spouse become sicker and sicker until they draw the line and seek help. My body felt like it must be dying, so we packed up and went back to the emergency room. At this point, we were still going to the American doctors on the base. Again, after hours and hours of waiting, prodding, and poking, we were told that they could not find any answers to explain my pain. No answers. No hope. No direction. Sonograms revealed a cyst on my ovary, but nothing abnormal to the doctor. The gynecology exam gave them no answers for the extreme abdominal pain. The blood results showed nothing in my blood. When the doctors inferred that these symptoms were perhaps in my head, something I was making up for attention, I challenged them: "Aren't you concerned that I could not walk when I came in here? Don't you want to find the reason for why I could not walk?" To which they replied: "Well, you can walk now." Yes, three rounds of morphine later, I could walk out of the hospital. While strong painkillers are not my preference, I was in a world of hurt, so I took them in order to pretend that this living hell was not happening to me. I think I resorted to the medical drugs more to numb my feelings of hopelessness than for the actual physical pain. With painkillers in hand, a heart drained of hope, and a wife that was higher than a kite, my husband packed us up and returned us home.

That solidified my new routine: I was home on painkillers, living a life mostly in bed, and still in so much pain as I watched the sun rise and set with no answers. To add to the frustration, the brain issues grew. I remember banging my head on the bathroom counter one night, my brain numb on one side, as I sat there and prayed that I wouldn't die. My thoughts were so fuzzy that I struggled to communicate basic sentences to my friends and family.

On a daily basis, my symptoms continued to change, causing my anxiety to grow. My throat began to feel like a huge lump was in it, and at times I struggled to swallow. Have you ever had to tell yourself over and over, "Swallow, swallow!"? What in the world? On a different day, I remember standing in the kitchen and feeling snakes crawling up and down my spine. Now it was getting completely crazy! At this point, to say that my mental status was not in a good place would be an understatement. Life was dark, and the darkness of feeling misunderstood can be a very scary place to live out. Some friends and family began to tell me that this was my new reality and that I must accept this as my life, but this only made the fighter in me rise up. By no stretch of the imagination would this ever be my reality. I knew that we would find the answers, but I just did not know yet where they would come from. I began to do my own research as I searched for answers. I searched for hope.

Google became my closest friend as I searched for every answer under the sun. I Googled things like, "numbness in face, numbness on left side, brain tingling, leg pain, abdominal pain." I wouldn't recommend Google as your doctor because I was usually only left with anxiety. "Maybe it was a stroke." "Maybe I will never walk again." "Maybe I have some rare disease." "Maybe it is Parkinson's like my mother told me." There wasn't much solace in searching the internet at this point in my journey because it only seemed to drive me down different horrible scenarios.

What I did find to be helpful was pulling out my *Essential Oil Desk Reference Book* by Gary Young and digging deeper into how the body works. I learned that most diseases come from a place of toxicity or mineral deficiency. I began to take minerals and supplements that I discovered that I might be low in. I also read up on how some herbs can help the body detox. I did not know much about detoxing, but I started with little changes. Since I was spending so much time in bed, I decided to begin watching the recorded essential oil classes that my mentor, who happens to be my naturopath and friend in Dallas, would send me each month. I was behind in my viewings, and I decided that, now more than ever, I needed the education. I began watching class after class, and if I could handle taking notes, I did that too. My friends and family were looking out for me and sent me research from all directions. I was desperate for answers, so I took the time to read everything and watch anything that anyone would send my way. Most of the research was helpful to some degree, but I began to realize that I needed to filter. I could not spend hours listening to everyone or reading everything. I began to pray that God would lead me to the answers that I needed and shield me from ones that only caused anxiety.

One morning, when my day once again began being greeted with my entire left arm going completely numb, I decided that this madness had to stop. It dangled as if I had had a stroke. I could not put on pants, let alone pull them up and down to go to the bathroom. This madness had to stop. I had had enough, and because we were not finding answers from the American Military hospital, I decided to brave it and go to the local Japanese emergency room. I do not speak much Japanese, but God always shows up. We headed to the only local Japanese emergency room that we knew, and a friend met us there to help watch our kids. Experiencing a foreign hospital always presents a learning curve, but adding the use of socialized medicine to that made our learning curve into a definite curve ball. Navigating the paperwork, the vitals, the language barrier, and more was frustrating. I had been experiencing such a variety of symptoms, and not only was my body exhausted, but my mind was exhausted from trying to explain the laundry list of symptoms as well. I remember my husband standing in the ER doing his best to describe what I was feeling and how many doctors I had already seen, and as I watched, I lay there feeling exhausted, hopeless, and defeated. How could we communicate all of this to someone with whom we could not even speak the same language? The numbness that my brain was experiencing was now taking over my heart. I felt numb to the world of ever gaining my life back. I watched the doctors do their best to listen and comprehend what he was saying, but I had no idea what was getting lost in translation. I'm sure everyone could feel the frustration in the room.

At just the right moment though, my friend, who had planned to meet us there, showed up in the ER and quickly introduced me to a stranger who would soon become a very dear friend. You see, this woman just happened to be hanging out in the emergency room because her husband was upstairs recovering from a recent stroke. God put her there at exactly the moment that we needed someone for translation. Teresa is an American who is married to a Japanese man, so she speaks great Japanese. Having her in the room quickly helped dissipate the level of frustration because she was able to hear my story and then translate it back to the doctors. It wasn't necessarily easy though. Not only does translating symptoms take a long time, but it also takes a lot of trust to tell a total stranger your medical situation and hope that they are translating it correctly to the doctors. This night was long, but a beautiful friendship between myself and Teresa began to blossom. She was there with me for the entire process of several emergency room visits. I would love to say that the Japanese doctors were able to pinpoint what was going on, but after an MRI and sonogram on my stomach, we were again sent home completely stripped of all hope. How could I have so many symptoms and yet no one could pinpoint the issue? Not only was my left arm, brain, and face numb, but our hearts were numb from all the trauma, endless tests, and no answers.

Time kept going, but I felt trapped inside our home. When no one can tell you what is going on within your body, you begin to accept that this is your new "normal," and you learn how to live life with extreme pain and a head that is bewildered by all of it. My head was not right, and on the good days when I would drive, there were times that I would feel like my vision was blurry or that I'd had one too many drinks. I was slow to process a conversation, and communication was more than embarrassing because words would get all mixed up in my head when I tried to articulate a thought. My equilibrium was off, and my spatial awareness was nonexistent. In order to not feel embarrassed by my lack of cognition, I began to retreat from socializing. Doing so only led to feeling more trapped by my circumstances. Even so, deep within my soul part of me still knew there were answers. I knew that I could not give up the fight. That part of me refused to accept that this was my new "normal." I just had no idea where to turn next, so life continued on with some good days and some days that kept me flat in the bed.

At this point, all of our friends, both local and those back in the States, were very concerned. We had asked for an opinion from every doctor friend that we knew. However, even the best doctors cannot easily diagnose things over the phone, so though we were always left encouraged by their love and prayers, we still felt alone. The friends here locally did not know us well because we had just moved to this part of Japan seven months prior. We had previously been stationed in Iwakuni, Japan and we were now adjusting to living in Okinawa, Japan.

It takes time to make lasting friends, but God showed up with those that He knew would deliver the love that we needed. The ladies from our homeschool group had heard the stories from others about what we were going through, so they put together a meal train and showed up to take the kids to their events. They also asked if they could come pray over me. I will never forget those women. Each of them have incredible hearts, and they sat there and listened as I did my best to share my story. I could see the concern in their eyes and their desire to help fix all of it, but no one knew what to do or where to turn. I think that up until these new friends laid their own eyes on me, they might have questioned what was going on. Maybe this was a spiritual issue and that they could pray it out. Maybe this was an emotional issue and some good counseling could turn things around. I believe that prayer works 100%, but I also knew that there was more to this story that just had not yet been played out. Once these new friends saw me, I think they also knew that this story was not finished yet too. We did only what we knew was in our control, and that was to get on our knees and cry out to our God. They sat and prayed over me while overwhelming tears of gratitude fell down my cheeks.

It was during this precious time with these women that I also cried because our daughter's birthday was the very next day, and I was too sick to throw a party. That's when my new homeschool friends kicked friendship into high gear. They went immediately into "mom mode" and began planning a party. I love a good party, but when I had them tell me that I could not attend, my heart was crushed. How could I seriously be too sick to attend my own child's birthday party? Reality set in as I received the iPhone updates, sharing pictures of all the people who had gathered, the cake, the presents, and a daughter with no mom at her party . . . .

And here I was at home, barely able to walk to the restroom. How can a body be this sick without anyone knowing why? How long was this entrapment inside of my broken body going to go on? These questions ran through my head, but so did extreme gratitude for the beautiful friends that loved us enough to be the hands and feet of Jesus to us during a time of utter confusion and sickness. The hours that were spent praying over me, I believe, were the prayers that helped point us to the next right step.

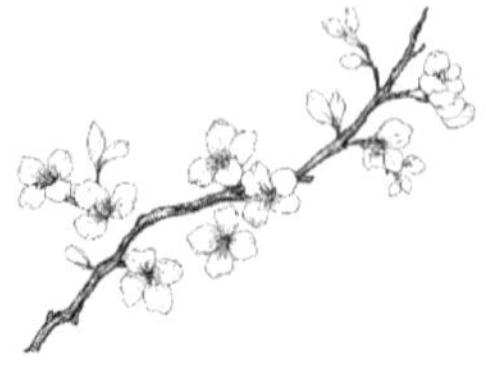

CHAPTER 2

Multiple Diagnosis

None of my symptoms were improving, so with my friends'
influence, I decided to go back to the local Japanese hospital, and
once again, my new and dear friend Teresa translated for me. She
was so very kind and gracious as she sat beside me and quoted
whole chapters of Scripture out loud as the doctor performed a
long and painful gynecological exploration. Between the cries of
pain, I thought, "I want to be like her—I want to comfort others in
pain with chapters and chapters of Scripture." The diagnosis was
pelvic inflammatory disease. Say what?? This seemed like a
desperate fabrication to me. Now, PID was not what I wanted to
hear, but to some degree, it was the very first time that I had an
answer of some kind, so despite my inner certainty that there was
no way this could be correct, I decided to take the treatment.

Have you ever had those moments when you know the
situation ain't good, but for some reason, it needs to happen? Much

later, I learned why God allowed this moment. You see, what do doctors in America use to treat a recent case of Lyme disease? They give you a huge dose of antibiotics. What did the Japanese doctors give me for this mistaken diagnosis? A massive amount of IV antibiotics. God works in mysterious ways, and sometimes those ways are extremely humbling on all fronts. Those antibiotics gave my body a little respite from the breakdown that it was having. That dose gave me a little reprieve, and at that point, my family and I needed it. For a few weeks, my symptoms calmed enough that I could function in some ways. I will never forget the feeling of excitement because I was able to make lunch for my children that day without having to sit down multiple times. This was a huge accomplishment and one that we all rejoiced in together.

All too quickly though, the pain returned in full swing. My nights were again full of my heart waking me after feeling like I had run five miles. Once all of the symptoms were back again, my husband began rubbing a series of essential oils every four hours up and down my spine several times a day. Although we had used oils in my bath water and a diffuser, this was the first time we began intentionally using oils in and on my body. The oils on my body would alleviate the pain for a while, but when it came back, it came back in all shapes and sizes. I would ask my husband to again layer the oils on my spine and this simply became routine because I found that it helped.

The oils that seemed to make the most difference were the oils that come in the Raindrop Kit from Young Living. These are all oils that help with blood circulation, lymphatic movement, and more. At this point in our lives, we had been using essential oils and herbs for our wellness routine for nearly ten years, so we naturally always gravitated towards them, but I'm not sure that we had been using them with such intentionality until this moment. To calm my racing heart during the night, I would apply two or three drops of Stress Away directly over the heart location.

Although the pain had returned with a vengeance, it was during this time that I began to realize that I did have some amount of control over how I was going to heal my body. I had been depending on the medical community; I thought they had all the answers. What I had forgotten was that even within the medical community, they are human. We humans don't always have all of the answers. We humans are flawed and sometimes make misdiagnoses. I knew the answers were out there, but at this point, the answers that lay within my reach were the intentional use of essential oils and prayer.

I do believe that God created us to function with a healthy mind, a healthy body, and a healthy spirit. When we are sick, none of those three are able to function clearly. Chronic sickness eroded away in all three areas until my mind was so clouded. I started to wonder if I was crazy. Maybe it was all in my head. My physical health was less than operational as I spent my days crawling from the couch to the bed. I was losing serious amounts of weight, and the lump in my throat was continuously there. The numbness would come and go. My spirit seemed so downtrodden. There is an emotional element to every dis-ease in the body. When you are left without answers as to why you are so sick, it takes a serious toll on your mental and emotional health. My mind, body, and spirit were at an all-time low, but I still had it within me to seek out answers.

My blood pressure was extremely low and I was at risk of passing out, so we knew that I needed to go back to the doctor. After numerous attempts to get answers from the American doctors, I decided to be brave and return to the Japanese hospital where they were willing to run more tests. I remember barely being able to walk to the restroom. The nurses could see that I was so sick, so they shuffled us off to the secret waiting room that had private little beds and a chair. While trying to walk to the restroom within this private area, a Japanese doctor who spoke clear English came up to me and asked, "Are you okay? What is wrong?" She waited until I was back on the bed and then came in and asked me to tell her my story. I was thrilled to have not only a woman that seemed to understand my woman's heart, but also one that easily understood my language. I did my best to quickly unpack my story. After listening, she told me that there was no way that I was leaving the hospital until I saw a neurologist. God always shows up. We had to wait such a long time that the hospital was closing up, when out of nowhere this same doctor delivered a man who couldn't speak English to us. She translated, I spoke, and he ran a series of neurological tests. To my total surprise, I failed the neurologist test and he told us I needed to stay in the hospital.

I was full of fear as they checked me into the hospital. The nurse then came to my bedside and apologized that the hospital was full to capacity. The only place that they had to put me was in the emergency room. I love the Japanese culture for so many reasons, but one reason is for their respect. They felt so bad that they couldn't provide a room that they tried to place me in my own room within the ER. When they pulled my wheelchair up to the tiniest room that resembled something out of a horror movie, I froze. I am claustrophobic and the size of that room was not going to help my mental status. Teresa translated my fears to the nurse. They then decided that it would be better to place me on a gurney and set me out with all of the rest of the ER patients. That's when the screams and moaning began from all around us. We quickly began second-guessing our choice. Maybe a small jail-like cell would be better than experiencing everyone's trauma. I refused to let my husband leave my side, which meant that he was given a chair that was made for tiny people and we placed our children in the care of others. After hours of trying to sleep sitting up he chose to curl up with me on the gurney. To say that it was a very long night would be an understatement.

While staying the night, the doctors performed yet another CAT scan and an MRI. The doctors did not like the results that they found. They had serious concerns about two spots that were showing up on my brain. They did not speak English so they looked up the translation and wrote the two possible diagnoses down on paper and handed it to me. We of course quickly Googled the terms written on the paper and then tried not to panic. We also sent a screenshot to one of our doctor friends in America, and he verified that neither diagnosis was a good outcome. He didn't have much encouragement, so he told us to pray that it was the lesser of the two evils because one was not as bad as the other.

The next morning the specialists arrived, and we were able to watch them contemplate as they went over and over my results. They delivered the news that whatever spots they were looking at were not what they initially thought they might be, but they had no answers as to what the spots were. Their only prescription was to come in and be checked weekly at the hospital. I still hate that I had so many CAT scans run on my body, but when you are desperate, you do whatever can possibly provide answers. We left that morning with the residue of nightmares and the feeling of defeat, but also extremely thankful to be out in the fresh air.

And so I began my weekly scheduled appointments with my newly assigned Japanese doctor who spoke broken English. Socialized medicine has its ups and downs, but I would say, after the hours and hours that I spent waiting at the local hospital to see my Japanese doctor, I am not a fan. I would have an actual appointment, but that did not seem to mean much. I still had to wait for hours, which for me only meant more time away from my children who were at home waiting to know if their mommy was going to get better. The waiting rooms were packed full of people.

In addition, there was a learning curve to the process. I had to check myself in, take my own temperature using a thermometer that everyone else had also stuck under their armpit, take my own weight and blood pressure, turn in the entire report to the nursing station, and start waiting. My faithful friend, Teresa, would show up and sit with me. She would always ask for a complete update and then would begin praying. After her prayer, she would share with me what she found so interesting about my symptoms. She did her best to help me connect the dots. At times, we would have to wait so long that I remember sleeping on benches in the waiting room. Now, if you know me, you would know that I am very aware of germs. Sleeping on a stranger's bench just isn't something that I would normally ever do. I knew that I was so sick because this became a weekly habit.

Each week, I would share with my doctor my latest symptoms: the lump in my throat that made me feel like I was struggling to breathe or swallow, the pain in my stomach that continued to double me over and led me to limit my nutrition to simple things like liquids. My brain struggled to process, and my communication would sometimes become a stutter. My ability to read became blurry, and my left arm would lose sensation from time to time. The pain from my knees down to my toes kept me from being able to walk correctly, and often I chose to crawl rather than walk. My blood pressure remained dangerously low. My heart would randomly race at high speeds. The doctors asked me several times if I had been in the mountains, rivers, or waterfalls. Finally, they asked me if I had been bitten by anything. It was then that I remembered the random pimple on the side of my rib cage, so I pulled up my shirt and showed them the location of the pimple, which I later understood must have been a bite. I will never forget the look on the doctor's faces when I quickly yanked up my shirt. It wasn't until that point that I began to make a connection. They studied the leftovers of what used to be a bite and now looked like a scar on my skin. No one had an answer, but this was a moment when I began thinking.

These weekly appointments slowly provided answers to some of my symptoms. I learned that I had a cyst on my ovaries that had burst, explaining some of the abdominal pain. It appeared that I had a cyst on my liver that had also burst. Additionally, I had a cyst on my thyroid, thus explaining why my throat felt swollen and I struggled to swallow. With every single one of these results, the doctors would tell me that it's normal to have cysts from time to time. I did not understand everything at the time, but I knew that it was never God's intention for a body to be filled with cysts and be told that it was "normal." I later learned that cysts are a sign of inflammation in the body and that Lyme sufferers are particularly prone to getting them. Inflammation in the body leads to dis-ease. Simply eating a diet that lessons the inflammation in the body would have been a great idea for me, but no one mentioned that.

During one of those weekly appointments, I had three doctors standing over me just baffled, and then a diagnosis came: Guillain-Barré Syndrome. I'm sorry, what? How do you even say that?

They then told me to be thankful because it could be so much worse. I could be like the people upstairs in the hospital who are now on feeding tubes and cannot swallow on their own. I was informed that it would take a year for my body to heal, but the doctors never really told me how to begin the healing. They told me that I would need to rest a lot. We had no idea what to do with the diagnosis, but it did send me on a mission to learn what Guillain-Barré Syndrome was and what to do next.

I have a mother who suffers from the damaging effects of Parkinson's disease. I would love to say that calling my mother to find comfort or support is what happened, but that would not be the truth. Instead, I was told, "Welcome to your new reality. Isn't it awful?"

With every fiber of my being, I refused to accept that a nasty disease would tear my life apart at the ripe old age of forty. I had a lot of time on my hands, as the bed was where I spent most of my days, so I began doing my own research, and search I did.

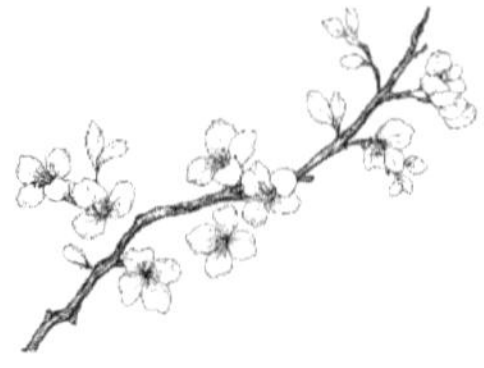

CHAPTER 3

Research

As more and more people told me to welcome my new reality or to just rest, I learned that others were not going to give me the validation that I desired. My road back to wellness was going to be one that I chose, and if others did not agree, I quickly learned that their opinions were not going to define my journey. I refused to accept that I should be grateful or welcome in my new "normal." I of course went home and Googled "Guillain-Barré Syndrome." I read every single article that I could find. Some of the research did comfort my soul because, to some degree, the symptoms and scenarios matched the hell I was going through. I devoured story after story of others sharing how their worlds fell apart by the devastation of Guillain-Barré. As I researched how to heal my body naturally from this syndrome, I began finding similar stories of people being told they had autoimmune issues. This reminded me that the doctors had tried to tell me that I too had autoimmune issues. I had also never heard of this before, so thus began my search into what exactly is an autoimmune issue. I was my own best advocate, and that meant I had to spend hours searching and praying for answers. It was a lonely place to be.

At this point, I spent nearly every waking hour researching either on the internet or digging into my *Essential Oil Desk Reference Book*. I wanted to understand the body. How does it work? What contributes to health and what contributes to illness? As I have said, throughout my ten years of learning about how to support our family's wellness via the use of essential oils, I had the opportunity to attend monthly meetings to further my education. While I was busy doing my current research, I was reminded of the numerous educational videos that had been sent to me that I had not yet taken the time to watch. Thankfully, I had kept a file with every single monthly video tucked safely away on my computer. Now, more than ever, was the time to sit and listen to education on numerous topics from gut health, toxin-free living, hormone balance, emotional wellness, and the list goes on. I began taking notes in a notebook that I kept beside my bed. I was amazed at how each time that I spent reading, searching the internet, or watching videos I was able to connect information with something else that I had learned. The pieces were ever so gradually beginning to come together.

As I listened to my children playing, cooking, doing school, doing chores, and living life, I would sit in my bed and cry. I knew that they deserved more. They deserved a mother who was actively serving them and living life with them. There were times when I would crawl down the stairs and lay on the couch just to feel like I was alive and an active participant in their lives. They needed me to smile and tell them that I was going to be okay. They could see right through me. They knew that I was in so much pain. I knew that I was valuable enough to fight for myself. I knew that my life was worth fighting for, but I just didn't have all of the answers. The kids were watching me at every single turn in this process. They saw me crying in frustration. They saw me crying from the intense pain. They saw me crying because I was living in fear.

It is my prayer that through their experiences they have learned many lessons, lessons of courage and grit, of strength and dependence on our God. I hope they internalize the lesson that no one has complete authority over you to tell you how you will live or what you must accept. I hope they see and believe that each of them is valuable to our God and their health is always worth fighting for, even if that means taking drastic measures or being called "weird" or "extreme."

I have no doubt that as they grow up and reflect on that time in their life, they will be able to share their own lessons that they learned, lessons that I am not even aware of, but my prayer would be that each lesson deepened their faith in the one true God. When you are young, your parents are your world. I'm sure that to them it felt like their world was being turned upside down. It wasn't fair that their mom had to miss homeschool co-op, piano recitals, swim meets, birthdays, gymnastic practices, and so much more. They needed me to be the parent, and during this time it seemed like the roles were reversed. I could not stand this role-reversal, and it needed to stop, so I continued to search for the answers. Life needed to return to normal—not in a year or a decade or even a lifetime, but now, while my children needed me—so despite the fact that I really couldn't communicate well, read well, or handle the pain well, I endured, sucked it up, did my best to pretend like I could handle life, and continued my research.

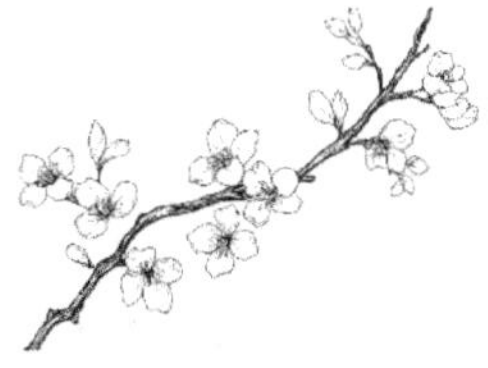

CHAPTER 4

Kampo

In order to function, I chose to take the doctor-prescribed pain medication. I knew far too much about the damage that it was doing to my liver to continue on this path, but I also knew that the kids needed their mother. I felt like a fake because I am the friend that tends to be referred to as the "crunchy one" in regard to health and wellness. Taking strong narcotics was necessary temporarily, but I didn't want to keep putting my liver through that. I continued to use essential oils up and down my spine, on my feet, in my body, in the bath, and in the diffuser, but I needed something more. One day, I was sharing my story and my desire to ditch the narcotics with a friend. She shared with me that she had a local Japanese friend who could point me to a Kampo Pharmacist who was about an hour south of my home. I had never heard of Kampo medicine, but I was miserable, and desperate times call for desperate measures. Within twenty-four hours, I had the location

41

of the local Kampo pharmacy. I had no idea what I was getting into, but the kids and I both knew that the emotional state that the narcotic pain medication seemed to place their mother in was not how any of us wanted to live. We all wanted something else to work, so we packed into the van and drove south to find this pharmacist, praying that what he had would work.

We drove up to our intended location to find that it resembled something of a Japanese version of CVS or Walgreens pharmacy. I think we were all relieved that it wasn't a dark alley with a witch stirring her cauldron. The pharmacy was full of everything from deodorant and toothbrushes to toilet paper and bandages. Our eyes scanned from left to right. We didn't really know what we were looking for, so I went up to an employee and asked, "Kampo?" She pointed to the right side of the store and led us over to the correct department. This is where things always get tricky when you have a need but don't speak the local language. You're never sure how what comes out of your mouth will be translated. Thankfully, the kind lady behind the counter spoke enough English that we could make things work. She told me to sit down and fill out a few pages of information. The two pharmacists wanted to know my exact symptoms and diagnosis. I did my best to fill out the form, and afterward, they asked for me to verbally explain what had been going on and for how long. When I shared the diagnosis of autoimmune and Guillain-Barré Syndrome they nodded and responded with, "Ay." I'm not sure how that translates to English, but when I hear Japanese friends say that, it translates to me as,

"Oh, I understand. Really?" I told them that the local Japanese hospital had given me the diagnosis, and when the pharmacists seemed to understand, I found comfort. They told me that they had helped other people before with this same diagnosis. We went back and forth for quite some time as I explained what I had gone through. They seemed very sympathetic and kind. The two of them went behind the counter and began pulling out different herbs that they believed would help. While we anxiously waited, the kids were doing their best to remain patient. I think they explored every aisle in the store and visited the bathroom numerous times. They were such troopers to be on this journey with their mom. I was just praying that not only would whatever I was about to purchase work for the pain, but that we would get home safely. This was the farthest I had been away from home alone with the kids in months, and I was not only nervous to be in an unfamiliar part of the island, but also nervous that I might not be able to think clearly enough to return us home. While we waited, I prayed for every detail of this journey to turn out well for all of us.

After what seemed like forever, one of the pharmacists came to the counter with a bag of herbs that were all packaged up for me to take home. She wanted to make sure that I understood everything. Even though I still did not understand Kampo medicine, I chose to sit there and listen to her directions. She told me how to boil these herbs and then drink them before bedtime as a tea. She wanted to make sure that I knew what I was drinking, so she took the time to print off a list of every single herb that was now in my daily tea regimen. This is one thing that I have come to appreciate about the Japanese culture: you may have to wait for an extended amount of time for services, but it's simply because they are going above and beyond to take care of you. She graciously printed this list out and carefully went over all of it with me.

At one point in the tea conversation, I thought I heard the word "donkey skin." My brain was muddled, and my Japanese wasn't fluent, so I kept assuring myself that she was surely not saying "donkey skin." My twelve-year-old son was also doing his best to help me by processing the words himself, but he could not keep his thoughts inside of his head. He leaned over my shoulder, got down in this sweet lady's face and asked very firmly, "Are you saying donkey skin?" To which she replied, "Yes." The three of us locked eyes and shrugged our shoulders. I was so desperate for healing that even donkey tea didn't sound all that awful. She assured us of its numerous health benefits and continued with her explanation of the instructions. I had no idea what our donkey tea mixture was going to cost us, but I learned at the checkout counter that a monthly supply would run us around $200. I reminded myself that healing can be worth a great deal, so I gathered my patient children, paid my bill for the newly acquired donkey tea, and loaded up the van. We drove home with expectant hearts and exhausted souls.

That first night the family gathered around the stove in curiosity and hope while we all waited expectantly as mom brewed her tea. Would this turn things around? Had mom just lost her mind? Would this help with the pain? Had we just wasted $200? The tea became our new normal. The nightly aroma that filled our house was a mixture of cinnamon, clove, donkey skin, and CBD. In order to cope with our unanswered questions, we all just had to make it a family joke that mom was brewing her donkey tea. After two nights of my donkey tea, I became a believer in whatever these herbs provided, because, for me, the tea brought the sleep that I so desperately needed. The incredible thing about the body is that it was made to heal itself when nourished the right way. One of the ways to heal is with good, deep rest. When the body is sleeping, there is so much going on in regards to healing. Finally, I was sleeping, and this rest sure made a difference in my emotional and mental state.

Since I was finding rest and the pain had lessened enough that I no longer had to rely on narcotics to alleviate the pain, I decided that I should learn more about Kampo medicine. Kampo medicine is a traditional Japanese medicine that combines therapeutic methods and medical herbal systems that originally came from China. I learned that 80% of Japanese medical doctors use Kampo. It includes most of the traditional Chinese modalities such as acupuncture, massage therapy, diet, and herbal medicine. At this point, I was only using herbal medicine and having my husband massage oils into my feet and spine. So, in some regards, we were on the right path in using Chinese medicine, but we were only using pieces of it.

Although I have not searched in America, I would think that if one wanted or needed to seek out a Kampo pharmacist in America that they could find one. Traditional Chinese medicine seems to be more easily accessible these days as people seek different avenues for healing and wellness. I would highly encourage others to seek Kampo as a means for wellness. I was able to slowly begin to walk again; my joint pain was still there, but the level and intensity of the pain came down to a functional level. The whole family will forever be grateful for the leap of faith that we took in seeking out the Kampo doctor.

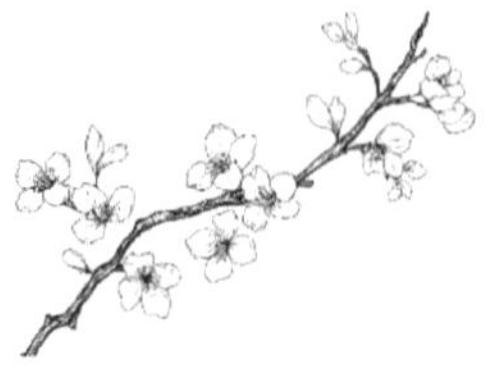

CHAPTER 5

Lyme

The more I slept, the more I was able to think and pray clearly. I continued on my journey in educating myself on living with Guillain-Barré Syndrome. As I searched, I found something that made me stop dead in my tracks. Lyme disease is often misdiagnosed as GBS. The wheels began to turn. I had that bite on my rib cage. I had a tick burrow into my thigh back in my twenties. Does Lyme settle in the body and hide? Does Japan have Lyme here? The questions just kept coming, but my symptoms fit way too easily into what Lyme disease looks like, so you had better believe that at my next appointment I asked the Japanese doctors the question, "Could this be Lyme disease?" I was quickly told that Okinawa doesn't have Lyme and that my symptoms couldn't be Lyme. They seemed adamant about it. I continued my weekly doctor's appointments for a while longer, but my herbs were working and my strength was returning. Although I wasn't healed,

I was better, and that's all the doctors seemed to be looking for. They told me to rest and wait a year for total healing, then released me from weekly appointments and encouraged to come for monthly check-ins.

I began my own research on Lyme disease in general and also found out that back in the 1990s, Japan declared that they did have Lyme disease here. The doctors had told me that maybe Lyme was on mainland Japan, but not here in Okinawa. How in the world could one think that Lyme could be on the mainland of Japan, but not here on the island of Okinawa with all of the daily boats that go back and forth? I will never understand that theory. I learned that Lyme doesn't just rely on ticks to transfer the disease. It can now be transmitted via rats, mosquitoes, fleas, and spiders. I just could not grasp how one could believe that this disease could not also be on this island. This is when I began to realize that mentioning Lyme disease seemed to bring up division within the medical community, but I had yet to uncover why this would be.

Because my symptoms seemed to be improving and the local doctors did not seem to be of help, I decided to discontinue going to my monthly doctor appointments. I no longer felt scared of the unknown symptoms, and I no longer felt dependent on the visits to the hospitals to guide me to answers. I will never forget the feelings I had as I walked myself to the car alone while leaving the hospital for the last time. So much of my story had happened within that foreign hospital. So much of my unraveling had happened with those people, and now I no longer seemed to need them. I still wasn't sure what I needed or where I would be turning next, but I had this strong sense that this was no longer where I needed to be. There was a certain amount of grief that I felt after so much health trauma, but there was also so much gratitude. Despite all of my fears, God always showed up in every ER visit, in every long doctor appointment, in every MRI or CAT scan. He never failed to provide me with the exact nurse, doctor, translator, or friend who could calm my fears and encourage me that I was brave enough to get through this. As I walked to my car, it was almost dusk and there was a sense of eeriness because the atmosphere of the hospital is a little dark, but no matter what I felt, I was leaving the darkness of sickness behind. The next chapter of my story was ready to unfold, but I had no idea what was ahead.

With a regimen of herbs and oils, many of my weird symptoms began to occur with less frequency. I was still slow in movement. Slow in strength. Slow in speech. Extremely slow in thought processing. I was also sensitive to light, and noises that most people could normally handle would feel like megaphones in my ears. Embarrassingly, there were times when I would have to leave social situations due to my lack of being able to process what I thought and have it come out of my mouth in a reasonable amount of time. When it did come out, my speech was sometimes slurred. Other times, I would leave because the noises or the lights just made my head hurt. The world I lived in was beyond lonely and scary, but I could walk and I had the strength to function at some levels, so things were "better." I hated living in what felt like a skeleton that was simply going through the motions. The family needed so desperately for mom to be healed, but at this point in my journey, "better" was more than good enough for me. I knew that I had improved, but something was still very much off. Not only that, but my mental health continued to suffer. I remember taking a family picture for Easter where everyone around me said how nice I looked, but inside I felt like I might just be slowly dying. I felt like a fake because I could not tell people that something was still so off. Everyone needed me to be well, so I continued to drink my donkey tea and use my oils so I could maintain at least at this level of health. I just kept reminding myself what the doctors had told me: I might need to wait a full year to see total healing. At this point, we were a short four months into the year. So trudged on with this new level of normal.

The days still found me spending hours in bed. I taught school to the children from my bedside. They would wake me and say, "Mom, I need help," or "Mommy, it's my turn to read with you," or "Mom, may I just sit here in bed with you and do my work?" Some people might say that I should have shuffled them off to school. There are times when my children might have been better off in a standardized classroom. All of those thoughts are valid, but that just isn't what we heard the Lord telling us to do. Life circumstances deliver, on a daily basis, far more than we can ever handle. Our family has personally experienced a family suicide, nearly losing our own child to salmonella poisoning, two near-death experiences for me from ectopic pregnancies, the loss of two babies, debilitating depression, financial stress, complete bedrest for pregnancies and so much more, but what we have also experienced is showing our kids up close and personal how we do and don't handle stress. They have seen our faith be challenged beyond measure. They have seen us wrestle with the things we know to be true and still put our faith into action. That's real life. That's where the rubber meets the road. They have witnessed me fight like heck to heal. They have learned a thing or two about health and wellness too because they have seen what sickness looks like and what health looks like. Those lessons are far more valuable than much of what they would have learned in school.

One day while in bed, I was reminded of a speaker who had recently spoken to our oils group about using essential oils to support hormones. In her introduction, she shared her story, a huge part of which was her journey with Lyme disease. I quickly looked up the video and watched her tell her story. Within twenty-four hours, I was on the phone with the guest speaker. We had so much to talk about. She was worried for my health and had no doubt that it was Lyme, but she insisted that I get on the next plane to the States. After an hour and a half, we decided that I would have to wait a long two months before heading stateside in order to be able to travel with my entire family. I was still too weak to imagine an international flight with four kids all alone.

During the waiting period, some days were good and some days were bad. I continued taking my daily herbal supplements and using essential oils internally, externally, in the diffuser, in the bath, and drinking my donkey tea. My body remained fragile, but I didn't want to believe it. In fact, I so badly wanted to be back in the game of life, that, one day, I went to play tennis with the family. Within less than thirty minutes, I broke my ankle clean through even though I had never broken a bone in my life.

This is where I have to push pause in my narrative and tell you that healing does not always happen immediately. In fact, it usually doesn't. I knew that truth on an intellectual level, but my heart so desperately wanted to be back to normal and to be able to care for my family again. I chose to put myself on the back burner and do what I thought would make everyone happy. Sure, going out to play tennis with my family also made me happy, but I knew better. I knew that I wasn't well enough or far enough in my journey of healing to jump into a game of tennis. I risked everything and drastically lost.

Up until this point in my life, I kind of laughed off the words "self-care." What did that even mean, and wasn't it rather selfish? My mysterious illness had knocked me flat, and just when I thought that I was on the road to recovery, the Lord allowed me to break my ankle, which only led me back to bed. As much as I didn't like it, I needed the pain medication to survive the first few weeks of life with a broken ankle. As I reflect on that time now, I can see how God was working hard to grasp my attention. I tend to be a Type-A kind of gal, and SLOW is just not in my vocabulary. I tend to operate from the mindset of, "Go big or go home." God had some important lessons for me to learn, but in order for me to listen, I feel that He had to knock me down in order to rebuild me. I had no idea what was ahead of me, but I soon discovered that I had so much to learn.

54

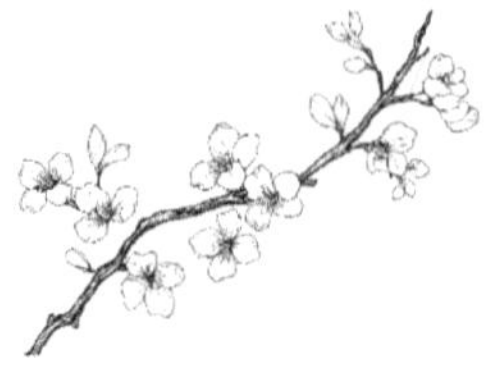

CHAPTER 6

Answers

Within two weeks of breaking my ankle, we boarded an international flight and headed to America in hopes of discovering the answers to our horrible months of darkness. Now, I do not recommend that anyone ever fly an eighteen-hour journey with a recent ankle break. It was a crazy, insane kind of tough for the entire family. Everything takes longer when your mother is in a wheelchair. It's also hard on a momma's heart when you have to watch your family struggle and there is nothing you can do to help. There were so many lessons that each of us were learning during this time, but it doesn't come across as a lesson worth learning when you are four years old and you need your momma. We were soon going to find our answers, but were we ready for what those answers meant for our family?

As soon as we arrived in the States, we visited a homeopathic doctor and I found myself in front of the electrodermal scanning machine. I will never forget when we found out that our thoughts were correct: I had neurological Lyme disease. If you know anything about Lyme, you know that multiple co-infections come along with it. My body was full of cat-scratch fever, several different kinds of Lyme, parasites, mold, and more. The tears were giant as they streamed down my face. I was so relieved. After being made to feel like a crazy person by the entire medical community, being hung up on when mentioning Lyme, and being told it was all in my head, I was validated by the certainty that everything I had experienced was tied to something going on within my body. Each pain that I felt, each symptom that I experienced, and each sleepless night all had a reason. My body had been trying hard to communicate with me, but I just didn't understand the message.

As the lady on the other side of the desk explained to me what was going on deep inside me and all that I needed to do to get well, my feelings of fear, exhaustion, and hopelessness set in. Sure, I felt validated, but how does one do all that needs to be done when there is no one to care for you? She encouraged me to begin thinking about not returning to Japan for a year. She knew that I needed to stay close to her office for follow-up care. We left with more questions and hearts that were very heavy. We had answers, but with them came more significant decisions.

I commonly get asked, "Did you get bit here in Okinawa or somewhere else?" That question is actually an extremely loaded one. Remember at the beginning of this story I had found that strange pimple on my rib cage? We will never know if my symptoms all began because of the recent pimple or from years ago when I had experienced a tick bite. Once I learned that Lyme disease can live dormant within the body, I began thinking back to an earlier tick encounter. When I was twenty-four, I had a tick burrow into my inner thigh and removed it with tweezers. I actually developed a red dotted rash on my inner thighs and forearms afterwards, but the doctor that I saw did not know what the rash was from. No one asked me if I had been bitten by something, and I never made a connection between the rash and the tick bite. I was told that it was something called petechiae, which is a skin rash. I now believe that it was my body's reaction to the tick. I did also become sick during this time, but none of us connected the dots.

Jumping back to 2016, I believe that "pimple" was actually a bite from something and that it was more than my taxed immune system could handle. My body had hit its limit, and that is why I quickly spiraled into a tailspin of one crazy symptom after another. I want others to know that ticks can be unbelievably small and you can be bit by one that you never see with the naked eye, but its bite can leave a nasty mark on your immune system. The bite on my rib cage was one that took me awhile to understand, but once I did, things began to add up and answers began to flow.

The next question that I began to ask was, "Why do some people's bodies instantly react to a tick bite but other people's bodies don't have symptoms for years?" This is a great question and one that I had to dig deeper into understanding. Our bodies are all very biochemically different, and we each have a different tipping point. A child's small body might instantly have a reaction within minutes of a bite simply because of their chemical makeup. Another adult may have a tick bite and not have a visible response for years to come. From what I have learned, it truly depends on the chemical makeup of each person and the strength—or lack thereof—in their immune system.

While sitting across the desk from my naturopath, Lisa, I took copious amounts of notes. I had less than a handful of knowledge about what exactly Lyme disease was, where it came from, and what my treatment would look like. I learned that Lyme is a bacterium and there are three different strands: Bartonella, Babesia, and Borrelia. Bartonella is a rickettsial bacterium. Babesia is a protozoa parasite of the red blood cells. I just happened have all three strands. None of them are good because they are spirochetes. They all act like magnets within your immune system. Spirochetes attack the immune system with a vengeance, creating space for other parasites, fungi, and viruses to come in and have a serious party. You can end up with all sorts of visitors, including mycoplasma, anaplasmosis, Cat Scratch Fever and Rocky Mountain Fever. That's pretty much what was going on inside my body. Every single pain, heart fluctuation, and weird sensation was not just in my head. I wasn't making up any of it.

Remember that lump I felt on my throat? The Japanese doctors told me that it was a small cyst and that it was "normal."

How does "normal" equate to me feeling such a large lump that I could hardly swallow? It doesn't. So many of the findings from the medical field were explained away to me as "normal." When I challenged the doctors with more questions, or if I tried to connect the dots myself and explain what I thought might be going on, I was met with blank stares and no answers. It seemed that they wanted me to accept "normal" and then walk away to live with the pains or ailments.

Sitting in the naturopath's office became a defining moment for me. The first appointment took hours as Lisa asked me one question after another. She asked if I had ever had Epstein-Barr, the virus that causes mononucleosis. Yes, I most assuredly did have it way back in high school. I remember being so sick and taking months or years to recover from it. That nasty virus loves to set up shop and hang around forever. Over twenty years later, it was still causing me trouble. I again allowed the tears to roll down my cheeks because I knew that I wasn't crazy each time I struggled to breathe and wondered what was going on. Mononucleosis doesn't like to leave the body, and some people fight for years to get rid of it.

The more I dug into understanding Lyme disease, the more I learned that there seems to be a dark side to the Lyme diagnosis that has nothing to do with the science. As I joined Google email groups and Facebook groups that were full of people suffering from the damaging effects of Lyme, I began to hear others' experiences. I heard story after story about the shame they felt because no one seemed to listen. People were struggling to find a doctor that would help them. How was this possible? How could so many people be suffering and yet find no one who would validate their symptoms, let alone diagnose what was going on? I learned that many doctors don't believe that Lyme is a legitimate thing, thus making it very hard to find someone who will diagnose and treat it correctly. I learned that in order to truly get the treatment that so many people needed, they had to find a Lyme-literate or an International Lyme and Associated Diseases Society (ILADS)-trained doctor. I had no idea what that truly meant, but I began to understand that a Lyme-literate doctor first believed in the existence of Lyme and therefore could help those who suffer from the devastating disease. In these groups, numerous people would post links which pointed me in the direction of learning and understanding the history of Lyme, opening even more doors to my research. I discovered that there most definitely is a dark side to living with Lyme and trying to find healing from it. Not only do few doctors even acknowledge its existence, but because of the controversial nature of its origins, even fewer people will treat it. If you'd like to follow my path, I've included some links to articles I found helpful in the resources section of this book.

I'll never forget the moment sitting in Lisa's office when I first learned that Lyme was my diagnosis. I looked across the desk at Lisa and begged her to give me a magic potion. My biggest question was, "How long until I am healed?" Of course, she couldn't give me the answer that I wanted, but she said that it generally takes about 18 months to get rid of all the bacteria in the body. I left her office that summer day with hope. I hadn't had a glimpse of hope for months. I had no idea if the bag of herbs and oils were going to heal me, but I had an ounce of faith. God tells us in His word that all we are called to do is to have faith as small as a mustard seed. Mustard seeds are crazy small. I had a little more than that, so I figured that I must be on the road to healing.

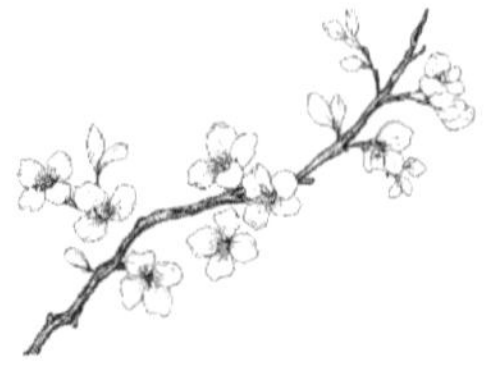

CHAPTER 7

Lyme Treatment

In addition to beginning research about living with Lyme, we began our prayers about staying in the United States or returning to Japan. We researched homes for rent in the local area. Unfortunately, we didn't have parents that would take us in and help with the children for a year while I crawled into bed and began to heal. To say we were burdened is an understatement. After much thought, research, and prayer, we decided that God didn't want our family to be separated. God allowed this to happen, so we walked in complete faith that we would begin the healing part of this journey as a family, in Japan.

The next big decision that we had to make was whether I would rely on homeopathic medications to rid myself of Lyme, use western medicine, or combine the two. I could work with both doctors and homeopaths an ocean away. I cried as I had to make this choice. I will never forget Lisa looking me squarely in the eye and saying these words, "Erika, I have only known you for these few short hours while I scanned you, but I can tell that you are a fighter. I would love to see you fight this without western medications. Now, the decision is yours, but I believe that you can fight this." Those words still bring me to tears today, because life is all about mindset, and so much of our health begins in our minds. Hearing those words spoken to me and over me made my spirit rise up. Yes, I am a fighter, and with the help of my family, I determined to beat this beast. I just had no earthly idea how I would do it. I left Lisa's office with a slew of herbs and homeopathic remedies though, ready to begin the next chapter of my story.

While in America, we also had friends and family come visit. We spent the next month or so visiting, catching up on doctor appointments for the kids, and traveling. Since the herbal treatments were likely to throw my body into detoxification, we decided not start the remedies until we were home in Japan.

In early August, we journeyed home with hearts full of so much fear. Living on an island in the Pacific and fearing that I could go backward in my health led to lots of anxiety for all of us, even my four-year-old. While in the airport, we had a funny experience that I will never forget. The airport security in Japan had to scan my wheelchair, and that made our little four-year-old nervous. He asked me what they were doing. I explained that they were making sure that I didn't have any bad stuff in me or on me. His response was, "Mom, I hope that they don't find out that you have worms in you!" I prayed with all my heart that the lady pushing my chair didn't speak English. I had no idea what to say or do, so I just laughed so hard until I cried. Teaching your kids about health and wellness is very important, but it can come back to bite you at just the right moment. We journeyed on and made it back to Okinawa with a mom still in an ankle boot, a suitcase full of herbs, and a stomach filled with parasites. We were a sight to see!

Once home, I began the detoxification process . . . and, boy, was it a process! I had no idea how much time in my day would be taken up with healing my body. While visiting with a friend at the park, she asked me to explain what I was doing each day. I shared my daily routine, but I didn't know how to answer her questions about my diet, and I especially did not like her suggestion about doing a daily coffee enema. I had heard about coffee enemas that summer while with a friend in Texas. I'm all about natural health, but this idea just seemed to take things to a whole new level. At this point in the journey, I wasn't ready to embrace such craziness.

Within two months though, I was lying on my bathroom floor learning to do a coffee enema. Never say "never," and always be ready to up your game. The first ten enemas were crazy-messy, and after that it just became routine. I did my research, learned where to buy the goods, and thus began my journey into a whole new side of detoxing. After a few months of doing this process daily, I learned that my body needed more in order to push out the heavy metals, cleanse the gall bladder, and purify the liver. Yes, I began doing two enemas back-to-back on the daily. What I quickly learned was that you can listen to podcasts, watch videos, listen to audible books, and even talk to friends while lying on your side in the bathroom.

The question you might be asking is, "Why? Why would you begin coffee enemas?" The answer is multifaceted, but it has everything to do with detoxing and cleaning out the gall bladder, intestines, and liver. These organs can accumulate toxic buildup, and when you ingest substances via the mouth, it takes a while before they can reach specific areas of the body. When substances enter the body from the other end, it's a much more direct route to cleaning out the system. People often misunderstand why you would do a coffee enema. In my case, they assumed that I was just trying to lose weight or remove constipation. That is an added benefit, but it wasn't the main reason I did them. I like to think of an enema as a way to wash the body. When you lie on the bathroom floor for twelve minutes, the compounds in the coffee are absorbed by your veins and have time to cycle at least twice throughout the body. I always enjoy the afterglow of feeling more clear-minded after doing my daily enema. As I used this process to help heal my system, it became a form of rebuilding that was happening within my body as I lay on the bathroom floor.

I doubt anyone would choose to heal on the bathroom floor. It's usually a place that is associated with being sick or maybe even with hanging over the toilet after having too much to drink. The bathroom floor is rarely associated with being the cleanest part of the home. But my bathroom floor is where I found myself, and this is where God and I learned so much together. My daily visits with the bathroom floor provided time to learn so much about the history of Lyme, and the more I learned, the more I wanted to dig deeper. One question seemed to lead me to another. Why did the military medicine hang up the phone on me twice when I asked if I might possibly have Lyme and could I be tested? Why didn't the doctors that I saw want to help me when I asked if it was Lyme? Where did this disease come from? Why do some people's bodies fall apart when bitten by a tick, and why do other people take years to show symptoms? These were just the beginning of the questions that I was asking, and so many of them were answered on the bathroom floor.

At this point in the book, you might be wondering how to do a coffee enema yourself. I will share with you a few pointers that I discovered, but I'm also gonna let you do your own research. Obviously, this is the story of how I healed my body naturally from Lyme. I am by no means a doctor, nor do I aim to be. I write to encourage you in your own journey.

Now, for the few tips that I learned: You must use organic coffee. There are coffee brands out there that are made only for enemas, but, for me, I found that any organic beans worked just as well. Steeping a pot of coffee every day can become daunting. I learned that I could steep a larger quantity at a time and then keep the extra in the fridge for up to a week. Doing this made the daily enema task more of a practical routine. I also learned that a stainless steel bucket was much more manageable to clean.

Speaking of cleaning, I found that keeping a household cleaner in the bathroom definitely helped speed up the daily ritual. Also, it is very important for the body to always produce its own bowel movement prior to doing an enema. I was advised to drink several ounces of water first thing in the morning before anything touched my lips. In doing so, I was waking my organs up and it nearly always produced a bowel movement.

During this time, I was also introduced to hair analysis. The hair on our heads is able to provide quite a bit of insight into what is going on within the body. Hair cut close to the roots gives scientists the ability to analyze which heavy metals one might be holding onto, which minerals one is high or low in, and how stressed the body is. As I was over an ocean from my practitioner and I wanted feedback on where my body was in the healing process, I chose to use this avenue. Thus, I began cutting a tablespoon of my hair close to the roots and shipping it to Arizona every six weeks or so.

It was also a whole new way of thinking. My results told me some of what I already knew, but they also revealed things that I didn't know. I learned that my body was extremely stressed, but then again, who wouldn't be stressed after all I had gone through? My adrenals were completely shot. I needed not only to detox but also to truly rest. The body has an incredible ability to keep our organs functioning as best as it can, and the ways that it does so are amazing. My body had been taking minerals and other resources away from where they belonged in order to keep me going. Adding hair analysis to my journey was a helpful turning point. I found it to be encouraging to receive regular feedback on my body's progress. I also needed the support as I had so much to learn, and although I was ready to throw in the towel, I couldn't. I had to keep going because I had four little kiddos that needed their mom back. So, I began to give my body healing foods and supplements based on what my hair analysis said that I needed. Thus began the next chapter in my Lyme journey.

Prior to the hair analysis, I had no idea that my body tends to be a slow oxidizer. That means that I don't process and absorb the nutrients from food very well. My body needed to receive the nourishment that was already beginning to break down. Doing so made it easier for my stomach to use the minerals from the food rather than just running the food right through my body without gaining any nutrition. I began filling my plate with 70% fully-cooked veggies at every single meal. God gave us a myriad of vegetables, but I had to be careful to avoid some of them. Eating nightshades was no longer an option. In addition, I only ate a protein twice a day. I had never eaten so many vegetables in my entire life. I could only have eggs once a week, red meat once a week, and the only fish I could have was sardines. Since my body was full of heavy metals, I had to avoid fish. There was a huge learning curve, and I would be lying if I told you that it was easy. There were times when I cried because I just couldn't eat one more bowl of veggies. I had to take time to read and learn. I had to let go of old habits and things that I had learned or come to believe were healthy. Healthy is good, but each of our bodies are biochemically different, and what is healing to your body might not be healing for mine. With this diet, what I did notice is that slowly, very slowly I was beginning to feel better.

I also learned that my adrenals were completely shot. The hair analysis showed that I needed zinc and lots of it. When your body doesn't get what it needs from the food that you eat, it begins to pull from wherever it can in order to support itself. Once you begin to give the body exactly what it really needs to function well, your body has to adjust. Imagine your adrenals being held up and supported by crutches. Imagine that when you begin to give the adrenals what they really need instead of crutches, the crutches get pulled from under the adrenals and the aftermath just ain't so pretty. I felt like someone had pulled the electrical cord from the outlet, and I was left to crawl back to my bed and sleep. The sleep was a better quality than I had had in years, but I needed lots of it. Feeling like this scared the you-know-what out of me. Was I going backwards? What if I never healed and was always this tired? My husband would slowly usher me back to bed and assure me that sleep was what I needed and that soon I would be better. I wasn't sure myself though. It broke my heart to find myself back in bed and away from our children. Adrenal fatigue is no joke, and if you find yourself there, I want you to know that there is hope.

The lymphatic system is a major detoxification system for the body, and when the system is clogged up, things that need to move out are not able to do that. Sweating every single day became the goal, and thus I also learned about the importance of the sauna. Not all saunas are created equal. I began visiting the dry sauna at the gym because that is what I had access to. Dry saunas heat up the skin from the outside and work inward, and this makes the detox process slower. With a near-infrared sauna, the light heats up the body from the inside out, which allows toxins to be drawn out from the organs deep within the body. I began by ordering one light from Amazon and aiming it at my stomach during my coffee enemas. Parasites hate the light, so this aided in cleaning out the intestines. Eventually, we ordered an at-home near-infrared sauna, and depending on the day, I would stand in the sauna for anywhere from twenty to forty minutes. I was shocked by how much better I began to feel. Between doing the daily coffee enemas and standing in the sauna, I became very familiar with the bathroom. Things were not only beginning to move within my lymphatic system and bowels, but more was moving within my heart and mind.

Hindsight is always 20/20, or so they say. Instead of saying this, what I like to say is that I am now a "Dot Connector." Going through my journey has taught me so many lessons, and one of them is the importance of asking really good questions and never accepting "no" for an answer when you feel deep within your soul that there is more. When I was so sick and desperate for answers, I left numerous doctor visits feeling hopeless and knowing that there must be more. My body didn't just become so sick overnight. It wasn't just because I had turned 40 and all the wheels were falling off. It was so much more than that. Now that I am on the other side of Lyme, I know more about why my body responded the way it did.

As a teenager, I was very sick. I had strep so many times that eventually the doctor looked my mother squarely in the eye and said, "If she gets tonsillitis two to three more times within the next year, then we will need to remove her tonsils." I had been so sick for so long that I knew that I would soon be having a tonsillectomy. Sure enough, at the age of eighteen, I celebrated my spring break with the removal of my tonsils.

I would love to say that the tonsil removal led to instant change within my body, but that wasn't the case. My body was so sick that my mother later confessed that she literally thought that I was dying. I tell you all of this to share that each time I was sick, the only thing the doctor knew to do was to provide me with antibiotics. No one ever dug deeper and explored more about why I continued to get so sick. Why did it always settle in my tonsils? Why could we never really seem to solve the problem? No one thought to try to heal any of my sicknesses naturally. It was just one antibiotic after another. Sure, antibiotics serve their purpose, and I am most grateful for their invention, but they also left a lasting effect on my digestive system. Overuse of antibiotics resulted in an overgrowth of Candida, which is a fungus that causes a myriad of symptoms within the body. I was left with a body that no longer absorbed nutrients from the food that I ate, had very few enzymes to process the food, and had irritable bowels that sent food right through me. Living life as a "normal" teen was not easy, but one that I still managed to navigate despite the fact that my nickname was "Poopy Pants." Those years of sickness left a permanent scar on my immune system that later reared its ugly head when my body had finally had enough.

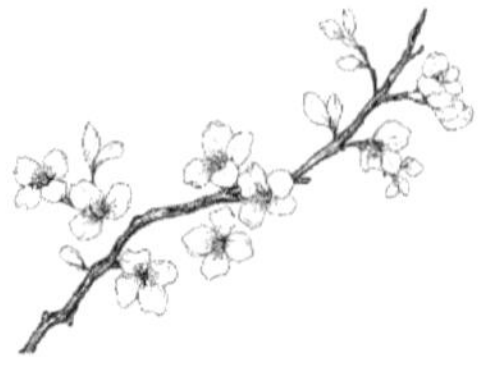

CHAPTER 8

Results

After a whole year of doing all I knew to do to fight for complete healing, I bravely left my family in Japan, flew over the Pacific Ocean, and walked into Lisa's homeopathic office. I so desperately wanted for my family to be there with me, but due to living overseas, unfortunately I had to visit alone. My dear friend Marisa refused to have me attend the appointment alone, so she journeyed alongside me and sat through the entire thing. She was my note-taker, and, man, did she not only take notes, but she verbally and emotionally helped me to process the information both then and later.

Because I had worked so incredibly hard at cleaning up my diet, resting, cleansing my body of toxins, taking all of my supplements, and taking all of my holistic herbs, I wanted desperately to see Lisa's face light up as she declared that she could no longer find any hint of Lyme or parasites left in my body.

But that is not what I saw. I could see that she was proud that the results showed her that I no longer carried the burden of Epstein-Barr. She was shocked by how much progress I had made, but I wasn't in the clear. Tears again filled my eyes and then fell down my cheeks. We all held hands that day in that small office and cried. We cried for the enormous progress I had made. We cried out of sheer exhaustion from the travel overseas to the appointment, from the hours on the bathroom floor away from my children in order to heal, from the money spent to order supplements, herbs, plane tickets, hotel rooms, and more only to learn that I wasn't out of the woods yet.

How could this be? How could I be doing all of the right things and still be fighting this disease? I didn't want to hear this at the time, but the answer is that God wasn't finished with me yet. You can do all of the "right" things, but if our God is working on something more beautiful than you could ever imagine, then no matter your fight, God won't allow complete healing until it is in His timing. I wanted so desperately to be declared Lyme-free, but God was doing something so much bigger, and He needed more time.

I left that day full of encouragement that I was on the right path and also discouraged that I wasn't fully done with this chapter of my life. I wanted so desperately to be done and I wasn't. Instead, I went back to the hotel with Marisa, and we raised a glass or two in celebration of all that our God had done up until this point and all that He was going to do to heal my body. We celebrated and declared that the magic potion that I needed was time and a whole lotta patience mixed with immeasurable grit. I knew that I had the grit, but I wasn't yet convinced that I had the patience.

If you would have told me that I would be visibly passing parasites a year and a half after diagnosis, I would have looked at you sideways. I will never forget seeing the evidence of the parasites in the toilet. I was so freaked out that I took a picture of it and also tried to measure it. When I got to over a foot long, I decided that I didn't want to know the truth–I knew enough. The whole thing left me in tears. I cried because of the dirtiness that passing something like that makes you feel. I cried because I had known for years that something wasn't right in two different places in my stomach. (Eventually, I learned that the pain was the parasite literally peeling off of the walls of my intestines as it was slowly dying.)

After my one-year appointment, my learning curve with parasites shot through the roof. I learned that I could only afford to eat fully cooked veggies. In order to get rid of the parasites and their eggs, I had to cut sugar and never entertain eating a fresh veggie. Cooking the parasites ensured that they were all dead before I ate them. I would love to say that this was the easy part of my journey, but it wasn't. For me, tackling Lyme was multi-faceted. I had more than Lyme to rid my body of, and I'm gonna guess that if you are reading this book, you do too.

I visited Lisa again a year later. Two years of utilizing walking as my only form of exercise, eating only fully-cooked veggies, kicking out nearly all sugar, performing two coffee enemas a day, and using daily supplements and herbs would surely deliver a Lyme-free diagnosis, right? I would love more than anything for the answer to be a joyful, "Yes!" But it wasn't for me. I'll never forget the bucket of tears that I cried as I yet again sat on the other side of that desk from Lisa and she praised me for my great progress, but she couldn't tell me that I didn't have this nasty bacteria still inside of me.

When we returned from America after that summer of travel and receiving my diagnosis, I had a strong sense that I was supposed to climb up into God's lap and listen. Part of my healing journey required that I learn how to rest. Rest has never been something that I'm good at, hence the diagnosis of adrenal fatigue. No matter how you are wired, I have learned that rest is crucial. I'll never forget the hair analysis dietitian telling me that I needed to rest at least twice a day. My response at that time was less than mature. I was like, "Have you heard of the four kids that I am raising, let alone homeschooling?" She asked if I had a friend with whom I could trade time in order to find some rest. I was frustrated because I was surrounded by Japanese people with whom I couldn't communicate. I couldn't imagine trying to ask them to exchange services so that I could find rest. The thought still makes me chuckle. Regardless, I found my own ways to rest as much as I could. I'm sure though that my journey to healing took longer simply because I struggled to make it all happen the way that it needed to happen. During this time, I had the overwhelming feeling that God wanted my utmost attention. I felt as if He wanted me in bed not only to rest, but also to really rest in Him and Him alone. What did that mean? I wasn't yet sure, but I knew that I needed this rest, so I did my best to rest in Him.

This rest took a lot of forms. Sometimes it looked like me closing the door, closing my eyes, and falling asleep. At other times, it looked like me closing my eyes, but not my mind. I would remind myself that resting needed to happen, and I knew that stopping the movement of life for even twenty minutes would do more for my body than drinking another cup of coffee and pushing forward. Other times, it looked like me falling asleep amongst complete chaos as the kids cleaned up the kitchen after lunch. At other moments, it meant resting in bed while a child read their daily reading assignment to me. There were also moments in the sauna where I would lay there, nearly asleep, as I practiced breathing from my stomach and then pushing the breath out from my top down to the bottom of my toes. All of these moments taught me a lot about my need for rest. They also taught me about the importance of slowing down and embracing the precious moments that life delivers but that we tend to miss because we are so busy.

During this time of learning to rest and heal, I had a business opportunity presented to me. I had many previous opportunities to grow my essential oils business, but never had I considered myself worthy of the calling. At this point, it was the end of February 2017—one year after that first bout of shaking. I could have argued every point as to why I had no time, no energy, and no bandwidth for growing my business, but this time things seemed different. My dear friend, Marisa, told me that she was gonna give this training a shot, and that is all it took. I was off. I could not allow the friend who I had taught about essential oils to go off without me on some training that I knew nothing about. I made a crazy decision to pursue business growth right in the middle of healing myself of Lyme disease. Let's be honest though, was I healing myself or did our God have me on a much bigger journey that simply required me to trust Him to heal me and refine me in the process?

I had no idea the crazy ride that I was about to go on, but I do remember getting up in the wee hours of the morning and practicing my daily routine of yoga while watching my dear friends within the oil world train me on how to grow my business. One early morning turned into another, and before I knew it, I found myself sharing oils with everyone I met. Oils had been a part of our lives for at least nine years at this point, so I knew enough to be sharing about their life-changing effects, but my battle with Lyme opened another part of my heart. I wanted everyone to know that they too could pursue wellness. One training led to another, and soon, I found myself in Salt Lake City, Utah, because I had won the last training. I give God the glory because all I did was listen to the training and do what they said to do. I don't share any of this to toot my own horn. I share this because I believe that if I hadn't gone through Lyme disease, I wouldn't have been at a point where I was ready to listen. Using oils in our home for the past nine years had become normal to us, but during my struggle with Lyme, they became one of our lifelines. Lyme also slowed me down in enough ways that I finally had time to listen. I listened to what God had had in front of me for the past nine years. I had known about oils during that time, but I hadn't been in the mental space to believe that others would listen to me. I didn't believe that I had what it took to build a business. Once I slowed down and listened to the Father's voice though, I had what it took to share the benefits of natural health with my friends and family. I had no idea that God had so much work to do within this part of my life.

How did I find the time to conquer all the healing that Lyme required and also to build a business from the ground up? To be honest, I do not actually know the answer. I do know that I have amazing kids that also had a front-row seat to my healing process. They knew that their mom was slowly blossoming into a new person. They knew that the refining that was happening was something worth celebrating. They were my biggest cheerleaders. They knew the depths in which we had all been, and they could see that each day I seemed more and more refreshed, refined, and renewed. They were truly the wind beneath my wings, so I journeyed forward and did every single scary thing that was placed before me.

We all knew that God hadn't taken us through the deep valleys of loss, death, sickness, and fear for nothing. We all knew, as a family, that God was doing something so much bigger, so we all put our whole hand in the pile and cheered for the 6G Network. Wellness was something that we had all tackled together, and we all knew that the world deserved to know how to pursue wellness. It was during this time that we launched *Little By Little Wellness, LLC*. Because I was a homeschooling mom and one that was running the biz from a foreign country, most of the business had to be run when my family was sleeping. Business podcasts became part of my daily routine, next to reading the word of God. There was a rebuilding of not only my mindset but also the mindset of our entire family, and we were all on a journey to deep healing.

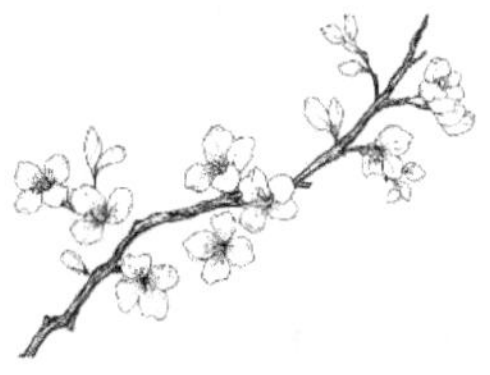

CHAPTER 9

All Things New

I wasn't out of the woods yet in regards to Lyme, but more and more God was uncovering false beliefs. I had to think bigger, and I was learning how. The unraveling of my limited beliefs was exhausting, but it was also extremely worth it. My bathroom moments were now being used to rebuild my mindset via the use of books on Audible, Facebook trainings, podcasts, and so much more. Two years prior, I had no idea that a person could attend a Zoom meeting while accomplishing an enema, but it is possible. I don't share this with you to embarrass myself or you. I share this because I believe that every single thing that happens to us in our lives has a purpose. If I hadn't slowed down long enough to listen, I wouldn't have heard that God had given me the gift of oils and also the freedom to build a business simply by sharing my journey. The slowing down allowed my mind to open and realize that there was so much more for our family.

People I interact with in my health business often ask for more details on what I did to heal my body so that they can take the same journey. Perhaps you're wondering the same thing. I hesitate to share this part of my story though because I know how I am wired. I tend to be the person that will hear how someone accomplished something and then believe that if I do the same thing, I will find the same result. That isn't always true. I never want to lead someone down the wrong path. My path had a purpose. My path took three long, grueling years. Yours might be longer. Yours might be shorter. I never want to lead anyone down a path that isn't right for what God has for them. I will share what I did with the hopes that you will take away what might be helpful to your personal healing journey.

As I've shared, once I was diagnosed with Lyme disease, I walked out of Lisa's office with a bag of homeopathic remedies. Because I had a host of parasites and numerous other viruses, my bag was loaded full. Homeopathy works differently than Western medicine. My body was full of "dis-ease," and our goal was to bring back me back to homeostasis. In order to do so, we had quite a journey ahead of us. Homeopathy gives the actual virus or bacteria to the body in slow doses and in minute forms. As the body receives these bacteria, it can build a defense against them. I took vials of Borrelia, Babesia and Bartonella in an orderly form. I did this for a year or two. The goal was to not just eradicate the active forms of the bacteria but also to target the biofilm. Don't get me started on the biofilm. The way I understand it is that biofilm is the nasty enemies that are dormant in my body, and any time they feel like causing a firestorm from within, they will. So, I took the vials for a lengthy period of time in order to leave no stone unturned. I also took tinctures of parasites and a few other things. I honestly don't remember every tincture that I was taking at that time because they were numerous—so numerous that I had to keep track with a written system just to ensure I took them all at the right time. I do know that another one was for the Epstein-Barr virus that had set up shop on my thyroid. Over time, as I learned what worked and what didn't, my Lyme journey transitioned from chaotically taking supplements and random wellness modalities into one of intentionality. Healing my body had become a targeted, intentional, full-time job.

With anything in the homeopathic world, the symptoms will often worsen before they get better. Once I began the tinctures and the vials, I knew I was committed and needed to be laser-focused. Quitting wasn't an option. The symptoms quickly escalated. The intense fatigue nearly took me down. I took every opportunity to rest that I could because I knew that in the resting, I was healing. I had to remind myself that even twenty minutes with my eyes closed, focusing on my breathing, was doing far more for my healing than continuing on in exhaustion. As the symptoms would rear their ugly heads, I had to continually remind myself that were simply "symptoms" and that they would quickly heal and be gone. Every single weird symptom of Lyme eventually went away.

For some Lyme sufferers, heat makes us feel a lot better. I lived on a subtropical island at the time of my diagnosis, which turned out to be a huge blessing. My lymphatic system was plugged up, and I needed to sweat to clean it out. The lymphatic system is one of the body's detox systems. We have several ways that our bodies detox via urination, bowel movements, lungs, and sweating. When any of your detox systems aren't functioning properly then the body isn't able to rid itself of toxins, thus causing further dis-ease in the body. A simple short walk or even just a moment sitting on the porch outside would provide instant sweat. As I researched healing my lymphatic system, I also learned the importance of the near-infrared sauna for sweating out toxins from deep within your organs, and we purchased one for our own home. I did my best to stand in the sauna on a daily basis. I say "stand" because the only place that we had to place the lights was at the back of our shower. During that time, I read, listened to podcasts, and did research. The length of my time in the sauna was determined by what my hair analysis reported. If I couldn't get into the sauna at home, but I was out and about for the kids' activities, I would use that time to drop by the gym and sit in the sauna for as long as time allowed. I was always amazed at how much better I would feel after sweating out the nasty bacteria.

In addition to using the sauna to address my lymphatic issues, I also did my best to walk for thirty minutes daily. Another way I added in movement was through massage. I found a lady in the neighborhood who was trained in lymphatic massage, and I went to her every week for a massage.

I sent my hair off for analysis every three months. I was always amazed at what my hair would reveal about what was going on inside of me. My hair would tell me what minerals I was high or low in. It also provided answers to which heavy metals I was or was not releasing. I was also able to see how I was progressing in my healing. Over the first six months of beginning my healing journey, I allowed myself very little room to get off track in my diet, sauna, supplements, oils, and homeopathy, and my hair showed the upswing in my health. Not only did my physical hair just look healthier, my hair analysis report reflected the progress. These changes were so dynamic that my progress was featured in the newsletter to encourage other clients who used this avenue for their own health journey.

Diet is everything, and now more than ever was I beginning to understand this. My hair analysis had revealed that I was a slow oxidizer. Years of a damaged gut required lots of attention to details in my diet. As I mentioned earlier, I ate fully-cooked veggies for three meals every single day. Seventy percent of my meal had to be veggies. I gave up all forms of grain starches for a solid year. Fully-cooked veggies allowed my body to not have to work so hard to break down the food. Eating like this also killed any parasites that came in the veggies. I ate very clean meats. No fish, since I was full of heavy metals. No raw sushi, since I was full of parasites. No sugar, as sugar feeds bacteria and parasites.

All of this was insanely tough. There were times that I would cry because I wanted to eat differently. I would cry at restaurants because there was nothing that I could eat. I would cry before social events because I wouldn't be able to eat what other people were eating. Eating so strictly is very lonely, but I began to find recipes that I could make ahead of time so that I had my own special treats. All of this was 100% worth it because I finally saw progress. There were certain veggies that I had to avoid because they would throw off my body's pH balance. At times, I would despair because I didn't want to learn one more facet of wellness—I just wanted to eat when I was hungry and not think about it. But then I would remember how far I had come and gather myself to journey forward.

I used oils in every single part of my journey. From diffusing for emotional support, to taking the Young Living Vitality Oils internally, to rubbing the oils up and down my spine, they were a part of my healing. I began watching weekly educational calls that would educate me on how to use the supplements and oils in more targeted ways, which then sped up my healing. I learned more about the importance of gut health and how the gut-brain connection is crucial to understand when pursuing wellness. I began consistently taking a probiotic and enzymes. My body desperately needed both. I believe that the use of oils is truly a lifestyle, and my journey through Lyme revealed to me how I needed to make it more of a complete lifestyle for myself and my family.

Fighting back against nasty parasites was a huge part of my journey and one that I now often find myself walking others through. For whatever reason, I was full of parasites. I would love to tell you that after one month of diatomaceous earth, I was cured, but that would be the biggest lie. I would love to say that these enemies were gone in six months, but they weren't. It took two years of actively doing all that I could to get rid of them. I would take two food grade diatomaceous earth capsules three times per day. After one month of taking it consistently, I would switch to the ParaFree supplement from Young Living for the next month. After a month of the ParaFree, it would be back to the diatomaceous earth and so on. During my daily coffee enemas, I would point a single near-infrared light towards my stomach to help push the parasites out. They don't like the targeted heat. I also took DiGize Vitality Essential Oil internally in capsules three times per day. This oil has tarragon and ginger in it, and parasites dislike both those herbs. To get in more tarragon, I sprinkled it on every single helping of cooked veggies. Staying away from sugar also helped to starve these enemies.

I love to run. I am not the fastest or the best, but I can throw on my shoes and find thirty minutes to an hour of free therapy simply by going for a run. During my time of healing, I was no longer allowed to run or do any kind of stressful cardio. For me this was like taking chocolate from a mom or cigarettes from a smoker. I use some serious cardio to burn through my thoughts. Exercise helps my sanity, and now I was not allowed to push. I felt like walking was for old people, but then I would remind myself of the time that I was too sick to even walk up the short hill from the beach to our home. Remembering this would cause me to be grateful for the comparative ease of a thirty-minute walk. Hard cardio would stress out my adrenals though, and I was busy trying to heal them. For me, I had to find humor in my frustration of not being able to run. When I would see a runner on the road, I would secretly have my own conversation with them by telling them how they were stressing their adrenals. Humor was my medicine for my lack of running. I am back to running whenever I feel like it, and every single time that I am out, I thank God for delivering me from being a woman who couldn't walk from the bed to the bathroom or from the couch downstairs to my room upstairs.

Because I was living overseas, I sent my hair off every six weeks and then, eventually, every three months so that I could tangibly measure my progress. If I had lived in the States, I would have gone back to Lisa's office every month and then every three months as my healing progressed. Finding a practitioner that can do electro-dermal scanning is the most helpful, and this is what Lisa does. I couldn't find one in Japan though. I would go back to the States on a yearly basis and sit in her office at an appointment for nearly three hours each time. We were always amazed at my healing but always challenged that there was still so much work to be done. She never allowed me to leave without encouraging me to journey forward.

These protocols seem daunting, and they were, but I am a fighter. I didn't want to have to pursue the western medical path if I could avoid it. I wanted to learn more about health and healing. I learned throughout all of these protocols that my body is strategic, incredible, and can heal itself when I make the choice to give it what needs and to stay away from things that don't aid healing. I had never before grasped this concept, and now I spend so much time sharing with others that no dis-ease in the body is your final sentence. It is not the end but only the beginning. What I find when I share is that other people have so many questions, but when I share the answers that I have found, their eyes roll back in their head. So many people don't want to find the grit from within, change their mindset, and begin their journey to healing. So many people want to live under the banner of sickness. It's an easy banner to wave—one that allows you to get out of so many things in life. It's a label that some people want to wear, but not me. I knew that God was doing something, and sickness was not where God wanted me to thrive. Yes, the days of crazy routines, meals, and therapies were exhausting, but slowly, ever so slowly, I found my way back to health.

As a person begins to lose weight, their body also begins to detox. I was focusing on detoxing every part of my body, and with it came weight loss. The human body has a way of storing toxins within the cells. Emotions that can be "toxic" are also stored in the cells. When we don't deal with those emotions in an appropriate way, our heart and brain find a way to push them to some organ that can handle the stress load. With the heavy metals, toxic emotions, toxins, fat cells, and other things that were coming out of me from the detoxing, I was a hot mess. My family will attest to that. I was focusing on detoxing the liver where lots of anger, bitterness, and resentment tends to be stored, and the rage was real. I have several moments that I am not proud of, and I have had to go to others and ask their forgiveness.

This part of my journey was shocking to me and one that I wasn't in any way prepared for. The rage that came out wasn't fair to anyone, especially to the little ones at my feet who sadly received the brunt of it. I would love to ignore this part of the healing because of the pain I feel from it, but I have to be honest with you. I would have wanted to know about this side of the journey. If someone had prepared me for it, I would have felt more normal—or at least been able to understand what was going on within my body. In the moment, when you are only seeing red and you don't normally function like this, it can be scary. I now understand more about how emotions play into overall wellness. There is 100% an emotional component to sickness, and I pray that you find a doctor that is willing to recognize this. The body is created to function in homeostasis, which includes the balance of body, mind, and soul. I don't believe that a body can be out of balance without each of those parts also being out of balance.

In doing all of these daily routines, God used each moment to speak to me and grow me. I so desperately wanted my healing journey to be celebrated at month eighteen of doing all of these protocols, but for whatever reason, that wasn't my story. I now believe that there was just a lot of work to be done from within. One huge part of the rebuilding was in my mindset. As Proverbs says, "As a man thinketh in his heart, so is he." From the time I was a small child, I had this way about me that others would call "bossy" or a "leader." For so many years, I'm not sure that I was truly walking in the purposes of my God. I'm not saying that I wasn't walking in His will for me, but I wasn't walking in the fullness of who He had created me to be. It was through the healing of Lyme that He had time to get my attention and show me that He has more for me. I slowed down long enough to realize that I could make time to take part in business trainings. He also undid some limited thoughts that I had allowed to define who I was and how I lived my life. Ever so slowly, I was becoming a new creation, and at times, it was seriously ugly. Some days, I felt like I was taking giant steps forward in learning to run a business in the wellness world of Young Living and also be a homeschooling mom, and then, at other times, I was beyond discouraged because I had no idea what I was doing. I began to think that I wasn't cut out for this. I would allow others to steal my sparkle for a short time, and then I would put myself back together again and get back at it. I had numerous times when I had to apologize for my lack of business savvy. Lyme was a time to further my education in regards to wellness and health. It brought me more gifts than I could have imagined—gifts that I get to share with others who are struggling and that God has used to bless our Young Living business.

I wish I could pinpoint all of the ways my mindset has changed, but I can't. I can say that I have allowed myself to dream again. I am also extremely aware of the words that we speak over ourselves and others. There is life and death in the power of the tongue, and I'm keenly aware of the choice of words that I speak now over myself and my children. I am also a believer that what we put out into the world comes back to us. I now take time to reflect on things when I don't like the circumstances or how people are acting around me. If I am putting out negativity into the world, then I can expect only negativity to come back to me. When I am pouring positive things into myself and conducting myself in a positive way, then I tend to find that positive people are drawn to me. Another aspect of my growth would be in communication. Communication is critical, no matter if it's with your spouse or a group of people. Learning how to run a business forced me to be precise and clear in my communication. Before Lyme, I always thought that I said too much, but I have learned that communication has so many forms and can always use some work. If I hadn't gone through my journey with Lyme, I am not sure that I would be running a business like I am today. I am thankful for the realization that I do have something to offer the world. I see the world differently. I see others differently. I see failures as opportunities for growth. I am forever changed, and I wouldn't give up the three years of crazy protocols for any of the lessons that I had to learn during that time in my life.

The day finally arrived when I sat across from Lisa as she declared that she could no longer find a trace of the Lyme bacteria in my body. When this moment occurred, I wept happy tears. We both looked at one another, tears streaming down our cheeks, and we praised our God. He ultimately worked out the healing, and we gave Him the glory for everything that had happened in the last three years. Some people told me that it would never come. Some people questioned all that I was doing. Sometimes I thought healing was impossible or questioned what I was doing. But at the end of it all, I was healed.

I stand here today and wish that I could look you in the eye. If I were eyeball to eyeball and belly to belly with you, I would speak so much life into you. You have what it takes to fight this nasty horrible disease. I know that it has taken pieces of your life, your health, your finances, your relationships, and so much more, but that doesn't have to define your future. For whatever reason, God has allowed this to be a part of your story, but it's not the end. I believe that the first step to healing is a positive mindset. You have to believe that you are worthy of being healed, and I will tell you that you are. You were not created to live in sickness. You have what it takes to pursue a clean diet, a healthy lymphatic system, taking the right supplements, and anything else that your healing journey requires. My business name became *Little By Little Wellness* because I believe that wellness is so multi-faceted that it's best to begin with one little step in the right direction, which will then lead to the next step in the right direction. Slowly, you will begin to see progress because today doesn't define who you will be in a month, a year, or three years from now. This little moment will soon be a story that you can share with people who are struggling, but you first have to look at yourself in the mirror and believe that your health is worth fighting for. You are worth fighting for. The tools to your healing journey will begin to unfold. I firmly believe this, and I cannot wait for you to reach out to me and share what avenues led to your healing. Your story is worth sharing. I write because I know the darkness. I know the doubt. I know the shame. I know that exhaustion. I know the level of pain. I write to tell you that you were created to rise up and fight, my friend. You were not called to live in the darkness of sickness. There is no joy there. First, you must rise up and begin to fight for your healing, and I promise that the joy will come.

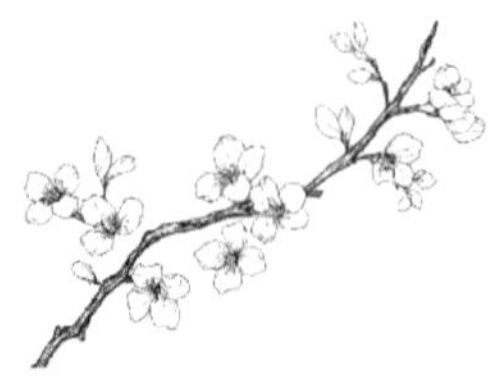

ABOUT THE AUTHOR

Erika Goering's tenacity for just about everything in life is contagious. She believes that life is meant for living to its fullest. In 2016, when Erika suddenly found herself bedridden with a sickness that no one could understand, she knew that there was so much more life to be lived with her four children and husband. With a deep faith and a passion for truth, Erika began searching for answers as to why her body had become so broken. Now, several years later, Erika resides in Virginia and continues to share the story of her battle with Lyme disease. Whether you are chatting with her at the local farmer's market, homeschool co-op, real estate auction, thrift store, or staging a property, you will connect with Erika's passion for wellness of mind, body, and spirit.

Follow her online at:

Website: goeringhomesllc.com

Instagram: @erika.goering

Facebook: Little by Little with Erika

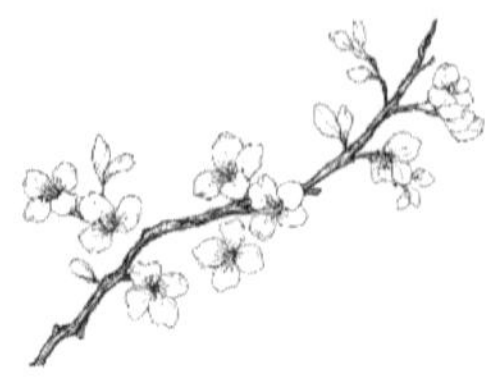

RESOURCES

GENERAL PRODUCTS
Almond Butter
Not being able to eat any sugar was difficult. I found that when I had a craving for something fun or sweet, I could curb that craving with a scoop of almond butter.
https://www.amazon.com/gp/product/B00AJ58FQM/ref=ppx_yo_dt_b_asin_title_o04_s00?ie=UTF8&psc=1

Diatomaceous Earth
Food grade Diatomaceous Earth was helpful to aid in ridding my body of the parasites. I would take this for 30 days at a time, two times a day.
https://www.amazon.com/gp/product/B07H451KK1/ref=ppx_yo_dt_b_asin_title_o08_s00?ie=UTF8&psc=1

Enema Coffee
It's important to use only organic coffee when doing a coffee enema. This product was what I used at first but later learned that as long as I was using organic coffee, it was fine.
https://www.amazon.com/gp/product/B00OVBGFZI/ref=ppx_yo_dt_b_asin_title_o03_s00?ie=UTF8&psc=1.

Enema Kit
I found that using a stainless-steel enema pot was far easier to clean than a bag.
https://www.amazon.com/gp/product/B0022V8G1A/ref=ppx_yo_dt_b_asin_title_o03_s00?ie=UTF8&psc=1

Enema Tubing

I also found it to be important to have extra tubing around the house to frequently replace the enema tubing (it eventually develops mold).
https://www.amazon.com/gp/product/B01MDS83EP/ref=ppx_yo_dt_b_asin_title_o03_s00?ie=UTF8&psc=1

Foot Detox Machine

I used the foot detox machine as often as possible to rid my body of the toxic load.
https://www.amazon.com/Cleanse-Machine-Vitality-Booklet-Brochure/dp/B00LFW6Y48/ref=ppx_yo_dt_b_asin_title_o03_s00?ie=UTF8&psc=1

Near Infrared Sauna

This is the company that I ordered my sauna from. I placed this in my shower and did my best to stand inside of it for around 20-40 minutes per day. Sweating daily is key in releasing toxins from the body.
https://creatrixsolutions.com/near-infrared-sauna-lamps/?fbclid=IwAR2tCAkeBXT6ZyXhuDLSF2DWYivx45l DKJ5PCGyOb7FkwkeopMYia7-4Wls.

Tarragon

I used organic tarragon as a seasoning on top of my fully-cooked vegetables. Tarragon is an herb that has been found to rid the body of parasites.

<u>YOUNG LIVING PRODUCTS</u>

Digestion support

Essentialzymes-4, Detoxzyme, and Life 9 are three supplements that aided in the absorption and digestion of my food. I needed all of the digestion support possible and found these to be very useful.

Emotional Support

Chronic illness is difficult, even without adding in the work of healing. I found that I needed a lot of emotional support. I used the oils that tended to help me on the emotional level. Those oils are Valor, Inner Child, Release, and Stress Away.

Immune Support

Thieves oil was a constant in my diffuser and topically on my feet to help boost my immune system.

Joint Pain

I used Peppermint, Basil, Panaway, and Wintergreen oils topically to help me deal with the intense joint pain.

Parasites

During the month that I would rest from the diatomaceous earth, I found that taking Comfortone daily seemed to help cleanse my gut.

Spine Massage

The oils that my husband would massage into my spine were Valor, Basil, Marjoram, Oregano, Wintergreen, Thyme, and Cypress

To order any of these young living products, go to www.youngliving.com and click on "Become a Member." Don't panic. No stress. At the next point you can choose if you would like to place a retail order or a wholesale order. It will explain the difference there. Go ahead and order whichever kit or products you're interested in. Place my member number, 958442, as the enroller and sponsor. Decide which shipping you would like. If you order over 100 PV, which is around $100, then you qualify for free shipping. Decide if you want to order monthly on our incredible program where you earn rewards points to cash in on products. Totally your decision. Checkout and send me a 💬 so I can begin to place a fun thank you gift in the mail. It's that easy. Thanks so much for choosing me 😊

PROVIDERS

Hair Analysis

This is the company that I used to evaluate my hair samples and then work through nutritionally balancing my body. http://drlwilson.com/

ILADS (International Lyme and Associated Diseases Society)

ILADS has a provider search on this website to find a doctor near you who is versed in treating Lyme. https://www.ilads.org/patient-care/provider-search/

Lisa Cox, EDS Certified Technician at Soteria Health Services

Lisa was instrumental in my healing. 3120 Hudson Crossing, Suite 4A, McKinney, TX 75070. Phone: (469) 712-7540

LYME ARTICLES

"Babesia Symptoms Can Be Deadly: A Family's Story" By Dr. Daniel Cameron https://danielcameronmd.com/babesia-symptoms-can-be-deadly-a-familys-story/

"Touched By Lyme: CDC Serves Up Same Old Wrongheaded Lyme Advice" By Dorothy Kupcha Leland https://www.lymedisease.org/touched-by-lyme-cdc-serves-up-same-old-wrongheaded-lyme-advice/

"What Are Lyme Disease Co-Infections?" By Dr. Daniel Cameron https://danielcameronmd.com/lyme-disease-co-infections/

"What to Know About Babesiosis, the Rare Tick-Borne Illness That Attacks Red Blood Cells" By Korin Miller https://www.prevention.com/health/health-conditions/a36607721/what-is-babesiosis/

CONNECT WITH ME

More information about a healthier way of life and some of my Lyme journey can be found on my YouTube channel at https://www.youtube.com/channel/UCpfOwo81Ylwgd95-36NNWpw

www.ingramcontent.com/pod-product-compliance
Lightning Source LLC
Chambersburg PA
CBHW070952250726
48663CB00002B/189